SIMPLY SIR DIET

3 in 1

How I Lost 110 Pounds by Activating the "Skinny Gene" and Going on in Eating My Delicious Recipes. Bonus: Weight Loss Project with Intermittent Fasting and Autophagy

Josie Kidd

Legal & Disclaimer

The information contained in this book and its contents is not designed to replace or take the place of any form of medical or professional advice; and is not meant to replace the need for independent medical, financial, legal or other professional advice or services, as may be required. The content and information in this book have been provided for educational and entertainment purposes only.

The content and information contained in this book have been compiled from sources deemed reliable, and it is accurate to the best of the Author's knowledge, information and belief. However, the author cannot guarantee its accuracy and validity and cannot be held liable for any errors and/or omissions. Further, changes are periodically made to this book as and when needed. Where appropriate and/or necessary, you must consult a professional (including but not limited to your doctor, attorney, financial advisor or such other professional advisor) before using any of the suggested remedies, techniques, or information in this book.

Upon using the contents and information contained in this book, you agree to hold harmless the Author from and against any damages, costs, and expenses, including any legal fees potentially resulting from the application of any of the information provided by this book. This disclaimer applies to any loss, damages or injury caused by the use and application, whether directly or indirectly, of any advice or information presented, whether for breach of contract, tort, negligence, personal injury, criminal intent, or under any other cause of action.

You agree to accept all risks of using the information presented inside this book.

You agree that by continuing to read this book, where appropriate and/or necessary, you shall consult a professional (including but not limited to your doctor, attorney, or financial advisor or such other advisor as needed) before using any of the suggested remedies, techniques, or information in this book.

Table of Contents

SIRTFOOD DIET Made Simple 17

Introduction.. 19

My Story...20

Let's Start the Journey!..22

Chapter 1: How the Sirtfood Diet Works.................................. 23

An Appetite for Fasting..24

An Energy for Exercise 24

Chapter 2: What Are Sirtfoods and Why Are They Special?....... 27

What Are Sirtfoods? 27

Who is the Diet Suitable For?......................................28

Benefits of the Sirtfood...29

Immune Health 29

Heart Health.. 30

Stroke... 30

Thyroid Health 30

Type II Diabetes.. 31

Kidney Health... 31

Autoimmune Disorders.. 31

Bone Health 32

Neurodegenerative Disorders....................................... 32

Obesity.. 32

Aging.. 33

Inflammation... 33

Stress... 33

What Makes the Sirtfood Diet Special?.............................33

Why the Sirtfood Diet is Different 34

Chapter 3: Sirt Diet and Fasting 37

Sirtfood Diet Phases... 37

Phase One...37

Phase Two...38

After the Diet Phase 38

Sirtfood Versus Fasting 39

Chapter 4: The Blue Zones 41

Chapter 5: Lose Weight But Not Muscle 45

The Science of Weight Loss 45

After the Weight Loss Plan 48

Sirtuins and Muscle Mass... 48

Chapter 6: The Scientific Studies Behind the Sirt Diet 51

The Sirtfood Pilot Study 54

Results 55

Chapter 7: Athletes and Famous People Who Follow the Sirt Diet
....57

Chapter 8: Over 20 Sirtfoods 61

Arugula 61

Buckwheat.. 61

Capers... 62

Celery 63

Chilies 63

Cocoa.. 64

Coffee 64

Extra-Virgin Olive Oil... 64

Garlic...65

Green Tea..65

Kale..66

Medjool Dates...66

Parsley..67

Red Endive...67

Red Onions...68

Red Wine...68

Soy...69

Strawberries..69

Turmeric..69

Walnuts...70

Dark Chocolate...71

Blueberries..71

Capers ....Errore. Il segnalibro non è definito.

Tofu...71

Chapter 9: Top Tips for Sirt Dieting *73*

Chapter 10: Shopping for the Sirt Diet................................... *77*

Chapter 11: Complete Four-Week Plan.................................. *79*

Chapter 12: Breakfast *83*

Strawberry & Citrus Blend..83

Grapefruit & Celery Blast..84

Orange & Celery Crush..85

Tropical Chocolate Delight...86

Walnut & Spiced Apple Tonic..87

Pineapple & Cucumber Smoothie.. 88

Sweet Rocket (Arugula) Boost.. 89

Sirtfood Mushroom Scrambled Eggs... 90

Blue Hawaii Smoothie... 92

Turkey Breakfast Sausages.. 93

Chapter 13: Quick Fixes..95

Honey Mustard Dressing... 95

Amazing Garlic Aioli... 96

Paleo Chocolate Wraps with Fruits.. 97

Vegetarian Curry from the Crock Pot.. 99

Chapter 14: Lunch..101

Greek Sea Bass Mix.. 101

Pomegranate Guacamole... 103

Chicken Curry with Potatoes and Kale.. 104

Mushroom & Tofu Scramble.. 106

Chapter 15: Super Salads...107

Coronation Chicken Salad.. 107

Spring Salad with Strawberry Vinaigrette...................................... 109

Rainbow Salad with Lemon Vinaigrette.. 111

Chapter 16: Speedy Suppers...113

Fried Cauliflower Rice.. 113

Minty Tomatoes and Corn... 115

Pesto Green Beans... 116

Scallops and Sweet Potatoes... 117

Citrus Salmon... 118

Mediterranean Paleo Pizza 120

Chapter 17: Easy Sirtfood Snacks *123*

Kale Chips 123

Moroccan Leeks Snack 125

Honey Nuts 126

Snack Bites 127

Herb Roasted Chickpeas 128

Easy Seed Crackers 130

Chapter 18: Top Sirt Desserts *133*

Chocolate Balls 133

Warm Berries & Cream 134

Chocolate Fondue 135

Mocha Chocolate Mousse 136

Walnut & Date Loaf 138

Chocolate Brownies 139

Pistachio Fudge 140

Spiced Poached Apples 141

Chapter 19: Smoothie Sirt *143*

Kale and Blackcurrant Smoothie 143

Strawberry & Beet Smoothie 144

Matcha Berries Smoothie 145

Grapes & Rocket Smoothie 146

Kale & Orange Smoothie 147

Chapter 20: The Sirtfood Green Juice *149*

Celery Juice 149

Orange & Kale Juice 150

Grape and Melon Juice.. 151

Sirtfood Green Juice 152

Conclusion *153*

SIMPLY INTERMITTENT FASTING FOR WOMEN *155*

INTRODUCTION *157*

CHAPTER 1: WHAT IS INTERMITTENT FASTING? *159*

BENEFITS AND SIDE EFFECTS OF INTERMITTENT FASTING........... 159

POSITIVE ASPECTS.. 163

NEGATIVE ASPECTS OF INTERMITTENT FASTING 165

CHAPTER 2: INTERMITTENT FASTING AND AUTOPHAGY *167*

HOW AUTOPHAGY WORKS 167

THE SCIENCE OF AUTOPHAGY 168

3 WAYS TO KICKSTART AUTOPHAGY 169

EAT LCHF...169
PROTEIN FASTS 169
TRY INTERMITTENT FASTING...169

CHAPTER 3: HEALTHIER WAY TO LOSE WEIGHT *171*

CAUSE OF WEIGHT GAIN 171

A HEALTHY AND BALANCED DIET 173

REGULATING YOUR METABOLISM... 175

HOW TO USE FASTING FOR WEIGHT LOSS 175

CHAPTER 4: TECHNIQUES OF INTERMITTENT FASTING *177*

KINDS OF INTERMITTENT FASTS AND BEST PRACTICES FOR WOMEN
.... 177

WHAT YOU NEED TO KNOW ABOUT HUNGER 179

SIDE EFFECTS AND CAUTIONS WHILE MAKING THE TRANSITION TO INTERMITTENT FASTING 180

HOW TO START INTERMITTENT FASTING 181
    LEARN WHAT YOUR NATURAL EATING PATTERN IS..............................182
    START WITH AN EASIER FAST TRANSITION 182
    LISTEN TO YOUR BODY AND KNOW WHEN TO QUIT 183
    EAT HEALTHY IN BETWEEN 184
    AVOID EXCESSIVE LEVELS OF SUGAR 185

CHAPTER 5: WHAT SHOULD YOU EAT AND WHAT NOT EAT.... 187

10 GREAT FOODS TO EAT 187

3 FOODS TO AVOID..188

FOODS RICH IN NUTRIENTS IDEAL FOR A FASTING LIFESTYLE 191
    LEAFY GREENS..191
    GARLIC..191
    POTATOES 191
    TOMATOES..192
    BROCCOLI 192
    CAULIFLOWER 192
    SUNFLOWER SEEDS...192
    ALMONDS 192
    BLUEBERRIES...192
    RASPBERRIES...193
    CHOCOLATE 193
    BEANS 193
    RICE 193
    TOFU 193
    SALMON...194
    SHELLFISH...194

CHAPTER 6: TYPES OF INTERMITTENT FASTING DIETS 195

THE 16/8 METHOD..196

THE 5/2 DIET METHOD...197

THE EAT STOP EAT METHOD 197

THE ALTERNATIVE DAY METHOD... 198

THE WARRIOR METHOD... 199

THE SPONTANEITY METHOD 199

CUSTOMIZATION TECHNIQUES 199

CUSTOMIZATION TECHNIQUE #1: ALTERING THE DURATION OF EATING
WINDOWS 200
CUSTOMIZATION TECHNIQUE #2: ALTERING DAYS................................201
CUSTOMIZATION TECHNIQUE #3: ALTERING THE TIMING OF MEALS 201
CUSTOMIZATION STRATEGY #4: ALTERING MEAL CHOICES....................201
CUSTOMIZATION STRATEGY #5: INCLUDE YOUR LIFESTYLE 201

CHAPTER 7: DRINKS TO HAVE AND AVOID WHILE INTERMITTENT
FASTING 203

3 DRINKS TO AVOID 205

10 GREAT DRINKS 206

CHAPTER 8: TIPS AND TRICKS FOR A SMOOTH TRANSITION INTO
INTERMITTENT FASTING AND FOR SUCCESSFUL INTERMITTENT
FASTING 209

STAY HYDRATED 209

AVOID BEING TEMPTED BY FOOD 210

RELAX YOUR MIND AND REST A LOT 210

ENSURE THAT EVERY NUTRIENT IS CONSUMED EFFICIENTLY 210

CONSUME FOODS HIGH IN VOLUME BUT LOW IN CALORIES 211

CHAPTER 9: WHO CAN DO INTERMITTENT FASTING AND WHO
CANNOT 213

EXPLORING THE PREGNANT CANDIDATE 213

EXPLORING THE UNDERWEIGHT CANDIDATE 214

EXPLORING THE CANDIDATE WITH AN EATING DISORDER........... 215

EXPLORING THE DIABETIC CANDIDATE 216

EXPLORING PROBLEMATIC CHARACTER TRAITS 217

CHAPTER 10: COMMON MISTAKES *221*

CHANGING YOUR DIET CONSIDERABLY 221

EATING IN EXCESS WHEN YOUR FASTING PERIOD ENDS..............222

CONSUMING LIQUIDS THAT YOU SHOULD NOT BE DRINKING 222

CHOOSING UNHEALTHY FOODS 223

CHAPTER 11: DOES INTERMITTENT FASTING HAVE DIFFERENT EFFECTS ON MEN AND WOMEN? *225*

INTERMITTENT FASTING AND FEMALE FERTILITY 225

INTERMITTENT FASTING DURING MENSTRUATION 226

WHAT IS PCOS? 227

BEST TREATMENTS & EXERCISES FOR PCOS...............................227

BEST (IF) TIPS ON HOW TO LOSE WEIGHT FOR PCOS 229

INTERMITTENT FASTING: PREGNANCY AND BREASTFEEDING.......231

THE ARGUMENTS IN THE FIELD: A GOOD IDEA OR NOT? 232

POSSIBLE DANGERS 233
LESS MILK! NO MILK! 233
NO ENERGY! 233
IF YOU'RE SICK, IT WILL ONLY MAKE THINGS WORSE! 234
OTHER CONCERNS: ANEMIA, LOW BLOOD PRESSURE OR SUGAR, ETC.. 234

WHAT METHODS HAVE WORKED 234
LOW-INTENSITY CRESCENDO METHOD 234
FLEXIBLE, SPONTANEOUS MEAL SKIPPING 235
ONE WEEK OUT OF THE MONTH 235
OVERALL TIPS 235

EATING RIGHT WHILE BREASTFEEDING 236

INTERMITTENT FASTING AND MENOPAUSE 239

DIFFERENCES BETWEEN THE YOUNG VS. OLDER WOMAN...........240

CHAPTER 12: SHOPPING LIST FOR YOU WHEN ON INTERMITTENT FASTING *243*

BEST FOODS & DIETS FOR PCOS 245

CHAPTER 13: MEALS PLAN FOR INTERMITTENT FASTING *249*

CHAPTER 14: SHARING INTERMITTENT FASTING WITH OTHERS *253*

CHAPTER 15: A BIT OF EXERCISE *255*

CONCLUSION *259*

SIMPLY AUTOPHAGY *261*

INTRODUCTION *263*

CHAPTER 1: WHAT IS AUTOPHAGY? *265*

DEFINITION 265

WHY AUTOPHAGY WORKS 266

AUTOPHAGY FOR HEALTH 266

1. EATING A HIGH FAT, LOW-CARB DIET 267
2. GO ON A PROTEIN FAST...267
3. PRACTICE INTERMITTENT FASTING 267
4. EXERCISE REGULARLY 267
5. DRINK A LOT OF WATER 268

TYPES OF AUTOPHAGY 268

1. MACRO-AUTOPHAGY 268
2. MICRO-AUTOPHAGY...269
3. CHAPERONE-MEDIATED AUTOPHAGY.....................................270

CHAPTER 2: WAYS TO INITIATE AUTOPHAGY *273*

EXERCISE.. 273

FASTING.. 274

DECREASE YOUR INTAKE OF CARBOHYDRATES............................ 275

AUTOPHAGY DECREASES THE RATE OF NEURODEGENERATIVE

DISEASES 279

AUTOPHAGY CONTROLS INFLAMMATION 280

AUTOPHAGY BOOSTS THE PERFORMANCE OF MUSCLES 280

AUTOPHAGY MAY ENHANCE THE QUALITY OF LIFE 280

AUTOPHAGY BOOSTS THE HEALTH OF THE SKIN 281

AUTOPHAGY ENHANCES YOUR DIGESTIVE HEALTH 281

FIGHT INFECTIOUS DISEASE 281

AUTOPHAGY CAN BOOST A HEALTHY WEIGHT 282

IT REDUCES THE DEATH OF CELLS 282

CHAPTER 3: ANTI-INFLAMMATORY DIET BASICS 285

MOST BENEFICIAL FOODS AND BEST ANTI-INFLAMMATORY

SUPPLEMENTS 287

    BLUEBERRIES 287

    AVOCADO 288

    COENZYME Q10 288

    GINGER 288

    GLUTATHIONE 288

    MAGNESIUM 288

    SALMON 289

    VITAMIN B 289

    VITAMIN D 289

    VITAMIN E 290

    VITAMIN K 290

CHAPTER 4: FOODS THAT REDUCE METABOLIC INFLAMMATION

... 291

CHAPTER 5: INTERMITTENT FASTING AND AUTOPHAGY 295

1. THE KETOSIS STATES 295

2. THE RECYCLING OF CELLS 295

3. THE 54 HOURS SHIFT 296

INCORPORATING INTERMITTENT FASTING 296

   1. BE PATIENT AND COMPOSED 296

   2. ALWAYS LOOK FOR A GREEN DIET......................................296

INTO YOUR WORKOUT PLAN... 297

CHAPTER 6: PRECAUTIONS TO TAKE REGARDING AUTOPHAGY

AND FASTING 299

   WHO SHOULD AVOID FASTING 299

   WHO NEEDS TO BE CAUTIOUS?.. 300

CHAPTER 7: INTERMITTENT WATER FASTING.........................301

CHAPTER 8: COMMON KINDS OF WATER FASTING..................303

   1. DRY FASTING.. 303

   2. LIQUID FASTING 303

   3. JUICE FASTING.. 303

   4. WATER FASTING.. 304

   5. MASTER CLEANSE.. 304

   6. SELECTIVE FASTING 305

CHAPTER 9: WEIGHTLOSS AND WATER FASTING.....................307

   LOSING WEIGHT FOR THE LOOKS 308

   LOSING WEIGHT TO GET HEALTHY....................................... 309

CHAPTER 10: INTERMITTENT FASTING COULD HELP YOU AGE

SLOWLY..311

   AUTOPHAGY LOWERS RISK OF NEURODEGENERATIVE DISEASE .. 312

   AUTOPHAGY IMPROVES SKIN HEALTH 312

CHAPTER 11: HOW TO FAST CORRECTLY 313

   EXPERIENCE AND DURATION 313

   HEALTH 314

NUTRITION AND HYDRATION 314

RELATIONSHIP WITH FOOD.. 315

CHAPTER 12: AUTOPHAGY, KETOSIS, AND FASTING 317

DOES AUTOPHAGY NEED KETOSIS?.................................... 317

MEASURE KETONES TO DETERMINE AUTOPHAGY........................ 318

AUTOPHAGY ON KETO 319

ARE KETONES THE BEST FUEL FOR BURNING FAT? 320

HOW KETONES ARE GENERATED.. 320

WHY YOU NEED TO MAKE KETONES YOUR MAIN FUEL 321

WHAT FOODS TO EAT TO PRODUCE KETONES............................. 321

IS IT POSSIBLE TO INDUCE AUTOPHAGY WITHOUT STARVING
YOURSELF? 322

CHAPTER 13: HYPERTROPHIC GROWTH................................... 323

CHAPTER 14: LONGEVITY AND AUTOPHAGY 327

CHAPTER 15: OXIDATIVE STRESS AND YOUR HORMONES....... 329

*CHAPTER 16: FINDING THE LONG-TERM AND SHORT-TERM
BENEFITS OF AUTOPHAGY 333*

IT CAN BE LIFE-SAVING 333

MAY PROMOTE LONGEVITY.. 334

BETTER METABOLISM 334

REDUCTION OF THE RISK OF NEURODEGENERATIVE DISEASES 335

REGULATES INFLAMMATION 335

HELPS FIGHT INFECTIOUS DISEASES 336

BETTER MUSCLE PERFORMANCE.. 336

PREVENTS THE ONSET OF CANCER 336

BETTER DIGESTIVE HEALTH 336

BETTER SKIN HEALTH 337

HEALTHY WEIGHT 337

REDUCES APOPTOSIS 338

CHAPTER 17: BENEFITS OF ONE MEAL A DAY 339

KEY BENEFITS 340

WEIGHT LOSS...340

SLEEP 341

RESISTANCE TO ILLNESSES...341

A HEALTHY HEART 342

A HEALTHY GUT 342

TACKLES DIABETES...342

REDUCES INFLAMMATION 343

PROMOTES CELL REPAIR..343

IMPROVES MEMORY 343

REDUCES DEPRESSION...344

CHAPTER 18: FOODS THAT BOOST AUTOPHAGY 345

GINGER 345

GREEN TEA 345

REISHI MUSHROOMS 345

TURMERIC/CURCUMIN 346

EAT PROBIOTICS! 350

CHANGING YOUR EATING HABITS 351

DEALING WITH OTHER PEOPLE... 352

CHAPTER 19: CIRCADIAN RHYTHMS AND AUTOPHAGY 355

CHAPTER 20: SLEEP OPTIMIZATION 357

CONCLUSION 361

SIRTFOOD DIET

Made Simple

THE ULTIMATE GUIDE WITH EASY AND DELICIOUS RECIPES TO LOSE 7 POUNDS IN JUST 7 DAYS BY ACTIVATING YOUR SKINNY GENE, BURN FAT AND FEEL GREAT

Josie Kidd

Introduction

Have you heard of a diet that can help you lose weight even if you continue eating chocolates, coffee, and red wine? How about a diet that claims to have the same effects as fasting and exercise without requiring its followers to do either of those weight-loss strategies?

Looking at its promises, you might think everything seems to be too good to be true.

Before deciding to write this guide based on my experience, I did a lot of research, and often the information I found was incomplete, and this produced even more confusion.

After finding a direction to follow that convinced me of its validity, I decided to try modeling the Sirt lifestyle in my daily life.

My goal in this book is to guide and encourage you through the most important information of the Sirt diet without feeling overwhelmed and intimidated.

"Simply Sirtfood Diet" was born for this reason.

I know what it feels like to struggle with being overweight; you are desperate, sad, and frustrated.

And it hurts!

But I want to tell you that change is truly possible.

I did a lot of diets, and I always failed my goal, and then for a long time, the fear took over, and I didn't want to try again.

But stop trying would have meant losing all of me.

My Story

I think that the change came in my life when I realized that the journey was made up of a path of personal growth and the right diet that did not strip me of some pleasures such as red wine or chocolate.

I have seen many other people have great results and maintain at the same time a good mood and motivation to keep going.

I grew up in a family that loves eating and cooking all the time, not just during Christmas or birthdays; any excuse is good for partying.

Moreover, they love fast food, pizza, and sweet drinks, ginger ale, or cola.

I didn't use to drink fruit juices or fruit smoothies, much less water.

My sister's weight and mine started to increase a lot during middle school, but the problems started in high school, when my classmates despised me and finding a boyfriend, a mate who accepted me for who I was, was impossible.

I tried all kinds of sports from volleyball to basketball to swimming... I hopelessly wanted to find something that would help me lose weight.

But no matter how hard I tried, I always ate a lot and badly and continued to gain weight; the more sports I did, the hungrier I was.

My self-esteem collapsed! I took shelter in my family, my few friends, and above all in food... they were my only consolation.

Yes, my family is always very happy, but it is also a family where 70% of them are obese.

After college, I didn't have many friends, however, I met a guy, Victor, who I dated for a couple of years and who later became my husband.

I tried many diets, and my life was like this; a few months at 176 lb. and a few months at 265 lb.

I really couldn't take it anymore!

The pregnancy didn't make things better, and Mindy's birth left me more than 55 lb.

My family doctor, given my desperation, recommended a gastric bypass, but I never considered it; I've always been terrified by surgery.

Besides, I was sure that somewhere there was the right diet for me and that I just had to find it.

So I started doing research and confronting many other people who, like me, could not lose weight and keep a healthy weight, and when I discovered the Sirt diet that activates the skinny body gene, I immediately thought that this was the kind of approach I wanted to start my new life with; no more unnecessary sacrifices and constant stress for my body!

I decided to start in April 2018, and after a year of sirt diet, I definitely lost and never regained 110 lb., and my life has completely changed for the better; every day I wake up grateful, happy, and with much more energy.

My success has led other people in my family to start a healthier approach with food, and they are discovering the sirt diet and are very happy with it.

Today my family and I are fully satisfied and united, we like to eat together, but we have learned to choose carefully the right foods.

No more junk food and sugar-filled drinks that make you addicted and damage your life.

Let's Start the Journey!

After all, how is it possible for anyone to lose 7 pounds in 7 days without having to spend your whole day at the gym or buying special foods and dietary supplements?

The Sirtfood diet attempts to emulate the advantages of fasting diets, but without any of the drawbacks. In this section, you will learn about the theory of fasting diets and how the Sirtfood diet cleverly achieves the same effect, but without any of the actual fastings.

Burning fat is what you might expect if you essentially start starving yourself, but another interesting effect of fasting is that your body switches from the replication of cells to the repair of cells.

The Sirtfood Diet is a food lovers' diet. You cannot expect people to eat the way you do it for the long term. The Sirtfood Diet is turning all of that on its head.

The benefits are all from eating delicious food, and not from what you don't eat. The better food you consume, the greater the rewards you enjoy. It also encourages us to rekindle the lost relationships of enjoying mealtime. Whether you're on a movie set, on a music world tour, or managing a bustling home, the business you keep connecting with as a family depends on what your daily life means. Meals are an event where all come together to enjoy the company of each other. That can be done easily with the Sirtfood Diet. Eat freely, without guilt. Knowing the food you eat feeds on your wellbeing. The meal plans are realistic and easy to follow while still delivering delicious meals. There's a real satisfaction to see empty plates at the end of a meal, and everyone is content.

It doesn't allow you to implement extreme calorie limits, nor does it involve grueling fitness regimens (although remaining generally active is a good thing, of course). And just a juicer is the only piece of equipment you'll require. However, unlike any other diet out there that focuses on what to eliminate, the Sirtfood Diet focuses on what to add.

Chapter 1: How the Sirtfood Diet Works

You may have known about the Sirtfood Plan previously - mainly since it was accounted for vocalist Adele lost 50lbs after the arrangement - however, do you know what it is? The eating plan characterizes the 20 nourishments that turn on your alleged 'thin qualities,' boosting your digestion and your vitality levels. It stipulates that you could lose 7lbs in 7 days. The eating plan will change how you do proper dieting. It might seem like a non-easy to use a name. However, it's one you'll be catching wind of a great deal. Since the 'Sirt' in Sirtfoods is shorthand for the sirtuin qualities, a gathering of classes nicknamed the 'thin qualities' that work, in all honesty, similar to enchantment.

Eating these nourishments, state the makers of the arrangement, nutritionists Aidan Goggins and Glen Matten, turns on these qualities and "mirrors the impacts of calorie limitation, fasting, and exercise." It initiates a reusing procedure in the body "that gets out the cell garbage and mess which aggregates after some time and causes sick wellbeing and loss of essentialness," compose the creators.

The sheer breadth of advantages that folks have experienced has been a revelation, all achieved by simply basing their diet on accessible and affordable foods that the majority of people already enjoy eating, which is all the Sirtfood Diet requires. It's about reaping the advantages of everyday foods that we were always meant to eat, but within the right quantities and therefore the right combinations to offer us the body composition and wellbeing we all so dearly want, which can ultimately change our lives.

An Appetite for Fasting

That takes us to fast. Consistently, the lifelong restriction of food intake has been shown to extend the life expectancy of lower organisms and mammals. This extraordinary finding is the reason for the custom of caloric restriction among some individuals, where daily calorie consumption is lowered by about 20 to 30 percent, as well as its popularized offshoot, intermittent fasting, which has become a standard weight-loss method, made famous by the likes of the 5:2 diet, or Fast Method. While we're still looking for proof of improved survival for humans from these activities, there's confirmation of benefits for what we might term "healthspan"— chronic disease decreases, and fat starts to melt away.

Yet current fasting programs could also place us at risk of starvation, impacting our wellbeing due to a decreased intake of essential nutrients. Fasting systems are also entirely inappropriate for large proportions of the populace, such as infants, women during breastfeeding, and very likely older adults. Although fasting has clearly proven advantages, it's not the magic bullet we'd like it to be. It had to wonder, is this really the way God was meant to make us slim and healthy? There's certainly a better path out there.

Our breakthrough came when we discovered that our ancient sirtuin genes were activated by mediating the profound benefits of caloric restriction and fasting. It may be helpful to think of sirtuins as guards at the crossroads of energy status and survival to better understand this. There, what they do is react to pressures. If nutrition is in short supply, there is a rise in tension in our cells, just as we see in the caloric restriction.

An Energy for Exercise

It's not just caloric restriction and fasting that activates sirtuins; exercise does too. Sirtuins orchestrate the profound benefits of exercise just as they do in fasting. Yet while we are urged to participate in routine, moderate exercise for its multitude of advantages, it is not the method by which we are expected to focus our efforts on weight-loss. Research shows that the human body has developed ways of adapting spontaneously and reducing the amount of energy that we spend while exercising, seven implying that for exercise to be a successful weight-loss strategy, we need to devote considerable time and effort. The grueling fitness plans are the way Nature intended us to maintain a healthy weight is even more questionable in the light of studies now showing that too much activity can be harmful— weakening our immune systems, harming the liver, and leading to an early death.

Chapter 2: What Are Sirtfoods and Why Are They Special?

What Are Sirtfoods?

Sirtuins are critical for our health, regulating many essential biological functions, including our metabolism which, I'm sure you know, is very closely connected to our weight. It's also a key figure in determining our body composition, such as how much muscle we build and how much fat we retain.

Sirtuin genes regulate all this and more. They're also integral in the process of aging and disease.

If we can turn these genes on, we'll be able to protect our cells and enjoy better health for a longer life. Eating sirtfoods is the most effective way to accomplish this goal.

Sirtfoods are all plant-based, and they have many more benefits, in addition to being sirtuin activators.

Our bodies require energy to operate, and the majority of this fuel comes from three primary macronutrients: carbohydrates, fats, and proteins. These macros largely control our metabolic system and regulate how the calories we consume get processed by our bodies. This is why most diets focus exclusively on micronutrition and require you to calculate calories.

Our bodies need more than just energy to survive rather than to thrive, however, which is why micronutrients are so important. They don't impact our weight as obviously as macros, but they are the foundations of our health.

Micronutrients, such as vitamins, minerals, fiber, antioxidants, and phytonutrients, are *supposed to be* consumed along with our calories. Unfortunately, in the Standard American Diet (SAD), they're in very limited supply.

When your diet is primarily made up of large quantities of red meat and processed meats, pre-packaged foods, vegetable oils, refined grains, and a lot of sugar, you will have an almost total lack of micronutrition.

Plant foods offer the most micronutrients per calorie consumed. Every edible plant has a unique nutritional profile, protecting you from an innumerable variety of illnesses.

Sirtfoods, and other plant-based sources of nutrition, give your body what it needs to stay young and disease-free, and, as an added bonus, this will help you remain at an ideal weight.

The original Sirtfood Diet encourages you to commit to a 1-week reset phase and then a 2-week maintenance phase where you rely heavily on the Sirtfood green juice for a significant dose of nutrition along with meals rich in sirtfoods. Once the phases are complete, to retain your health for the rest of your life, you will need to continue incorporating these sirtfoods into your daily meals.

The Sirtfood Diet is not a miracle cure, but if you stick to these recipes, you'll not just impress your taste buds, but you'll also enhance nearly every aspect of your health. You don't have to count calories or starve yourself to get the healthy, youthful body you've always wanted.

Who is the Diet Suitable For?

The Sirtfood Diet is suitable for: People with perseverance and discipline nutrition-loving people with background knowledge The Sirtfood Diet is not suitable for: People who have a hard time consuming only a few calories every day Smart tips for everyday life Many advisers reveal which other foods are suitable for the sirtfood diet and which other foods are combined with them. These can be helpful in order to better plan daily food preparation and thus make it easier. Because a comprehensive knowledge of sirtuins, their effects, and how to best integrate them into your daily diet increases your stamina.

Relaxation is also an essential part of the sirtfood diet. In stressful situations, the hormone cortisol is released, which, together with insulin, stimulates blood sugar levels and causes the body to feel hungry during periods of rest. Mainly due to the calorie reduction, one should avoid stressful situations in everyday life as much as possible. Small activities to balance out like a little walk in the fresh air can work wonders.

Benefits of the Sirtfood

Immune Health

We all know that the immune system is important; you learn about it early on in school. However, most of us never consider our immune health until we get sick, and by then, it is already partly too late. Unless we come down with a cold, the flu, or worse, a disease of some sort, we give little thought to this vital part of the body. But, at this point, all our immune system can do is damage control, trying to fight off the infection so that it doesn't kill us instead. We would be much better off if we instead focused on immune health all of the time so that we can prevent these infections from occurring in the first place. Think about it, would you rather have to try to fight off the flu once you already have it or avoid ever getting it in the first place? Of course, polyphenols can't take the place of vaccines, antibiotics, and other medicine, but they can greatly help you and strengthen both your immune system's ability to prevent infections and fight off ones you might come down with.

Heart Health

Oxidative stress, a leading cause of cellular aging, has been found to be a factor in both high blood pressure and heart diseases. Therefore, scientists in a 2004 study sought to learn if the polyphenols found in tea could help treat overall heart health by repairing and reducing oxidative stress. The results were encouraging, showing that when stroke-prone mice with high blood pressure consume either green or black tea, they are able to greatly lower both systolic and diastolic blood pressure. By the end of the study, the researchers concluded that the regular consumption of tea could protect against high blood pressure in humans.

Stroke

Sometimes referred to as a brain attack, strokes are extremely dangerous. While it deals with blood and many of the same risk factors of heart disease that can cause it, it is a separate category of cardiovascular health as it centers in the brain. What happens when a person has a stroke? A tear in a person's blood vessels or a blood clot results in the supply of blood to the brain is blocked off. There are two types of stroke. These are hemorrhagic and ischemic.

When a person experiences a hemorrhagic stroke, it is the result of blood ballooning into a pouch of the artery, known as an aneurysm. When this balloon of blood and artery bursts, it causes the surrounding tissue in the brain to be flooded with excess blood. Hemorrhagic strokes are more deadly, and even when a person does survive, their prognoses are oftentimes worse than those who suffer an ischemic stroke.

Thyroid Health

While we all frequently hear about the importance of heart, lung, stomach, and other organ health, the thyroid is frequently underappreciated by all but those who have a thyroid disorder. The thyroid is a gland and part of the endocrine system, which produces, stores, and releases hormones for the use of our cells. If it either under produces or overproduces these hormones, it results in a number of severe symptoms that worsen as they continue to get further away from homeostasis.

Type II Diabetes

While polyphenols have long been underestimated, a study published as early as 2002 did analyze the effects of polyphenols from green tea on individuals with type II diabetes. This is great news, especially since type II diabetes is the most prevalent, and the number of people diagnosed only continues to rise. The results were incredibly successful, finding that these polyphenols are able to increase glucose tolerance and reduce serum glucose levels. Both of these effects were great, but they only improved and increased over time as the rats consumed tea-based polyphenols on a more regular basis.

Kidney Health

Many people develop kidney (renal) disorders as they age, which is only worsened due to poor dietary habits, excessive alcohol, and other lifestyle factors. Thankfully, a 2007 scientific review found that polyphenols are able to affect the kidneys from injury, increase antioxidant defenses, and keep the renal cells functioning in a desired state of homeostasis. This was especially helpful in diabetic patients who frequently develop diabetic nephropathy of the kidneys, which was lessened due to the polyphenols. Lastly, the study found that when participants drank red wine, the undesired effects that alcohol frequently has on blood pressure were counterbalanced thanks to the protective elements of the polyphenols.

Autoimmune Disorders

There is a wide range of autoimmune disorders, over a hundred in total, which can all affect the body differently! This naturally means that the way polyphenols help each individual disorder will vary. However, the good news is that polyphenols, in theory, should be able to help every type of autoimmune disorder.

Bone Health

It is incredibly important to protect your bone health, especially as you age. People frequently develop osteoporosis at an older age, which results in bone deterioration and bone mass loss. Both of these result in an increased risk of fractures and breaks, which is why many people begin to break more bones when they fall as they age. Not only should the elderly be concerned about this, as some people develop bone disorders at a younger age. People who have taken or have to regularly take prescribed steroids should be especially aware of the risks, as one of the most common adverse effects of steroids is bone deterioration.

Neurodegenerative Disorders

There are many types of neurodegenerative disorders that can affect people of all ages. However, the most common and worrying for most people is Alzheimer's disease, as we never know if it is a condition our loved ones or we ourselves will develop as we age. It is especially concerning, as Alzheimer's disease is only growing in prevalence each year, with forty-four million people worldwide living with the disease. Thankfully, we don't have to accept that Alzheimer's may simply be inevitable. While we might be unable to prevent it in all cases, studies have shown that by eating a diet rich in polyphenols, we can protect our brain health and greatly reduce our risk of developing this devastating condition.

Obesity

Sirtuin burns fats quickly, and that's what makes this diet a great help for weight loss. When we study all the cases of successful sirtfood dieters, we can clearly see how well they fought against obesity. Adele is just one example, who has amazed the world with her 30 pounds of weight loss achievement using the sirtfood diet. So, anyone who isn't able to lose some extra pounds for whatever reason can switch to sirtfood and then can see the magic happening.

Aging

Aging seems like a threat to all when those wrinkles start appearing on the skin, and the person feels weakened inside out! Well, this magic gene sirtuin can also play its part in countering the effects of aging. It helps DNA to prolong its life and also aid in the repair process. Sirtuin is also responsible for apoptosis and leads to the formation of new healthy cells. This is the reason that people who are entering into middle age should consider doing the sirtfood diet so that they could effectively fight the possible signs of aging in the years to come.

Inflammation

What appears to be weight gain or metabolic inactivity is mostly connected to inflammation of both cells and organs in most cases. This inflammation is both the result and cause of several health problems. Sirtfood does not only prevent inflammation at cellular levels but effectively prevents it at the tissue and organ level.

Stress

There is one added advantage that higher sirtuin levels can guarantee, and that is the reduction in stress and depression. Research is still being conducted on the relationship between sirtfood and stress, but sirtuin is that element that can enable quick brain cell recovery and boosts brain activity by getting rid of all the unwanted metabolic waste. Efficient brain functioning then leads to a reduction in stress. So, this sirtfood diet can also help with stress relief.

What Makes the Sirtfood Diet Special?

Studies have related some of the foods recommended at the sirtfood weight-reduction plan with fitness benefits.

As an example, ingesting slight quantities of darkish chocolate with an excessive cocoa content may additionally decrease the chance of heart ailment and assist in combating irritation.

Drinking inexperienced tea may lessen the threat of stroke and diabetes and help decrease blood pressure.

And turmeric has anti-inflammatory homes that have useful outcomes at the body in preferred and might even shield against persistent, infection-related sicknesses.

In truth, most people are fans of sirtfoods have demonstrated fitness blessings in humans.

But, evidence on the health advantages of growing sirtuin protein stages is preliminary. But Research in animals and cellular strains has proven interesting effects.

For instance, researchers have pointed that expanded stages of sure sirtuin proteins lead to a longer lifespan in yeast, worms, and mice.

A few pieces of evidence show that sirtuins. May additionally play a position in decreasing irritation, inhibiting the improvement of tumors, and slowing the improvement of heart sickness and Alzheimer's.

Why the Sirtfood Diet is Different

The sirtfood diet gained publicity when singing star Adele hired a personal trainer and followed his instructions resulting in a weight-loss of 50 lbs. Chocolate and red wine made the diet plan sound appealing, but we all know in our hearts that uncontrolled consumption of chocolate leads to weight gain, so what makes the sirtfood diet plan different? Is it just another fad diet advertised by a celebrity?

Everyone knows how to lose weight: you simply reduce your calorie intake. When your body is running normally, it stores excess energy as sugar (short term) and fat (long term), but when you cut back on calories, this stops. Your body knows the food you're eating won't support you, and so it pulls energy from your reserves. Short-term immediate requirements come from your remaining stored sugar, and longer-term requirements come from the fat you had already stored.

The authors of the sirtfood diet think they've found it. Their diet plan is said to provide all the benefits of fasting or rigorous exercise without actually having to do either. The result is a change in eating habits that can easily be sustained on a long-term basis. But this seems too good to be true. What is a sirtfood anyway?

Exercise and fasting are both ways to "turn on" the effects of sirtuins, but heavy exercise regimes are simply not possible for some people, no matter how much they may want to be healthy.

Chapter 3: Sirt Diet and Fasting

Sirtfood Diet Phases

For every newbie, it is important to understand that the sirtfood diet does not start with a single list of ingredients in your hands. Its implementation and adaptation are more than mere selective grocery shopping. Every diet can only work effectively when we allow our body to embrace the sudden shift and change in food intake. Similarly, the sirtfood diet also comes with two phases of adaptation. If a dieter successfully goes through these phases, he can continue with the sirtfood diet easily. There are mainly two phases of this diet, which are then succeeded by a third phase in which you can decide how you want to continue the diet.

Phase One

The first seven days of this diet plan are characterized as Phase One. In this phase, a dieter must focus on calorie restriction and the intake of green juices. These seven days are crucial to initiate your weight loss and usually help to lose up to seven pounds if the diet is followed properly. If you find yourself achieving this target, it means that you are on the right track.

In the first three days of the first phase, a dieter must restrict this caloric intake to 1,000 calories only. While doing so, the dieter must also have green juice throughout the day, probably three times a day. Try to drink green juice per meal. The recipes given in the book are perfect for selecting from. Pick a recipe given in their respective chapters and pair each with green juices.

There are many meal options that can keep your caloric intake in check, such as buckwheat noodles, seared tofu, some shrimp stir fry, or sirtfood omelet.

Once the first three days of this diet has passed, you can increase your caloric intake to 1,500 calories per day. In these next four days, you can reduce the green juices to two times per side. And pair the juices with more Sirtuin-rich food in every meal.

Phase Two

After the first week of the sirtfood diet, then starts phase two. This phase is more about the maintenance of the diet, as the first week enables the body to embrace the change and start working according to the new diet. This phase enables the body to continue working towards the weight loss objective slowly and steadily. Therefore, the duration of this phase is almost two weeks.

So how is this phase different from phase one? In this phase, there is no restriction on the caloric intake, as long as the food is rich in sirtuins and you are taking it three times a day, it is good to go. Instead of having the green juice two or three times a day, the dieter can have juice one time a day, and that will be enough to achieve steady weight loss. You can have the juice after any meal, in the morning or in the evening.

After the Diet Phase

With the end of phase two comes the time, which is most crucial, and that is the after-diet phase. If you haven't achieved your weight loss target by the end of phase two, then you can restart the phases all over again. Or even when you have achieved the goals but still want to lose more weight, then you can again give it a try.

Instead of following phases one and two over and over again, you can also continue having good quality sirtfood meals in this after-diet phase. Simply continue the eating practices of phase two, have a diet rich in sirtuin and do have green juices whenever possible. The diet is mainly divided into two phases: the first lasts one week, and the other lasts 14 days.

Sirtfood Versus Fasting

This leads us to an enormous question: if sirtuin activation increases muscle mass, then why can we lose muscle once we fast? In any case, fasting also activates our sirtuin genes. And herein lies one among the huge drawbacks of fasting.

Bear with us while we delve into how this works. Not all striated muscle is made equal. We have two main types, conveniently called type-1 and type-2. Type-1 muscle is employed for longer-duration activities, whereas type-2 muscle is employed for brief bursts of more intense activity. And here's where it gets intriguing: fasting increases SIRT1 activity only in type-1 muscle fibers, not in type-2. So type-1 muscle cell size is maintained and even noticeably increases once we fast. Sadly, in complete contrast to what happens in type-1 fibers during fasting, SIRT1 rapidly declines in type-2 fibers. This suggests fat burning slows down, and instead, muscle starts to interrupt right down to provide fuel.

So, fasting may be a double-edged sword for muscles, with our type-2 fibers taking success. Type-2 fibers are what comprise the majority of our muscle definition. So, albeit our type-1 fiber mass increases, we still see an overall significant loss of muscle with fasting. If we could stop the breakdown, it might not only make us look good aesthetically but also help promote further fat loss, and therefore, the thanks of doing that is to combat the drop by SIRT1 in type-2 muscle cell caused by fasting.

Chapter 4: The Blue Zones

There are five areas of the world known as blue zones where the population is known to live longer than average. These are Okinawa, Japan; Sardinia, an Italian island; Nicoya in Costa Rica; among the Seventh Day Adventists in Loma Linda, California; and the island of Icaria in Greece.

All of these locations are noted to remarkable for the average life expectancy of their population, but the island of Icaria stands out the most. One-third of the population lives until they are ninety. But what is even more remarkable is their low cancer rate (20 percent lower than most), low rate of heart disease (50 percent lower than most), and an almost total absence of dementia. A recent (2011) study looked at the islanders of advanced years and found that just as elsewhere, they had many of the known risk factors for heart disease. Their age and successful aging appear to be due to a Mediterranean lifestyle and interesting diet, rich in olive oil, fruits, and vegetables. The islanders drink herbal tea every day in addition to red wine, and many of their preferred foods appear on the sirtfood list.

Studies of these "blue zone" diets have shown that natives of all these areas eat a diet with a much higher percentage of polyphenols than the rest of us.

One example of an outstanding sirtfood is cocoa. When cocoa is rich in polyphenols, particularly the flavanol epicatechin, it seems to provide protection from a wide variety of health problems ranging from obesity to cancer. Commercial cocoa, stripped of its flavanols (and hence, no longer a sirtfood), provides no such protection.

Something similar is evident in the diet of Indians. Cancer rates in India are lower than in most western countries, yet when they move to the US or the UK, the cancer rates in these populations increases. Again, there could be many reasons for this, but scientists are interested in turmeric, a spice used in most Indian cooking, which is known to be a sirtuin activator and is hence a sirtfood.

Scientists learned a great deal from studying the diet of those inside the "blue-zones," but what is even more interesting is what happens to those who move away. The fact that they invariably develop "western" disease profiles shows that genetics are not the reason for the blue zone inhabitants' good health.

SIRT1 and sirtuin proteins are accepted to assume a job in maturing and life span, which might be identified with the defensive impacts of calorie limitation. The case behind the Sirtfood Diet is that sure nourishments can actuate these sirt-intervened pathways sans the limitation, and consequently "switch on your muscle to fat ratio's consuming forces, supercharge weight loss, and help fight offing infection."

Alongside red wine, dull chocolate, berries, espresso, and kale, sirtuin-advancing nourishments incorporate matcha green tea, additional virgin olive oil, pecans, parsley, red onions, soy, and turmeric (a.k.a. phenomenal flavors and go-to solid treats).

There's some science behind the cases of sirtfoods' advantages, yet it's exceptionally constrained and rather disputable.

The science on the sirt boondocks is still very new. There are contemplates investigating the SIRT1 quality's job in maturing and life span, in maturing related weight addition and maturing related illness, and in shielding the heart from aggravation brought about by a high-fat diet. In any case, the examination is restricted to work done in test tubes and on mice, which isn't adequate proof to state that sirtuin-boosting nourishments can have weight loss or against maturing capacities in an absolutely real human body.

Brooke Alpert, R.D., creator of The Sugar Detox, says there's an ongoing effort to recommend that the weight-control advantages of sirtfoods may come to some degree from the polyphenol-cancer prevention agent resveratrol, often advertised as a component in red wine. "All things considered, it is difficult to devour enough red wine to get benefits," she says, noticing that she does much of the time recommend resveratrol enhancements to her customers.

Chapter 5: Lose Weight But Not Muscle

The Science of Weight Loss

Surely the diet will seem to work for certain individuals. In any case, scientific confirmation of any diet's triumphs is an altogether different issue. Obviously, the perfect investigation to think about the viability of a diet on weight loss (or some other result, for example, maturing) would require an adequately enormous example – delegate of the populace we are keen on – and irregular distribution to a treatment or control gathering. Results would then be checked over enough timeframe with severe command over puzzling factors, for example, different practices that may decidedly or adversely influence the results of enthusiasm (smoking, for example, or work out).

This examination would be constrained by techniques, for example, self-revealing and memory, however, it would go some approach to finding the viability of this diet. Research of this nature, be that as it may, doesn't exist, and we ought to therefore be wary when deciphering essential science – all things considered, human cells in a tissue culture dish presumably respond differently to the phones in a living individual.

Further uncertainty is thrown over this diet when we think about a portion of the specific cases. Losses of seven pounds in a single week are ridiculous and are probably not going to reflect changes to muscle to fat ratio. For the initial three days, dieters expend around 1000 kcal every day – around 40–half of what a great many people require. This will bring about a fast loss of glycogen (a putaway type of starch) from skeletal muscle and the liver.

Yet, for each gram of putaway glycogen, we additionally store roughly 2.7 grams of water, and water is overwhelming. So, for all the lost glycogen, we likewise lose going with water – and henceforth weight. Furthermore, diets that are too prohibitive are difficult to follow and bring about increments in hunger invigorating hormones, for example, ghrelin. Weight (glycogen and water) will therefore come back to typical if the desire to eat wins out.

As a rule, the use of the scientific technique in the investigation of sustenance is difficult. It is often unrealistic to do fake treatment-controlled preliminaries with any level of natural legitimacy, and the wellbeing results that we are often keen on happen over numerous years, making research configuration testing. Besides, considers in huge populaces rely upon shockingly shortsighted and guileless information assortment strategies, for example, memory and self-announcing, which produce famously inconsistent information. Against this foundation commotion, nourishment look into has a difficult activity.

Sadly, not. Sensationalized features and often hyperbolic features of scientific information brings about the apparently unlimited debates about what – and how much – we ought to eat, further fueling our fixation on a "convenient solution" or marvel fix, which in itself is an endemic social issue.

For the reasons sketched out, the Sirtfood diet ought to be entrusted to the prevailing fashion heap – at any rate from a scientific point of view. In light of the proof we have, to recommend in any case is, best-case scenario fake and even under the least favorable conditions deceiving and harming to the authentic points of general wellbeing procedure. The diet is probably not going to offer any profit to populaces confronting a scourge of diabetes, sneaking in the shadow of corpulence. As expressed plainly by others, uncommon diets don't work, and dieting all in all is certainly not a general wellbeing answer for social orders where the greater part of grown-ups are overweight.

By and by, the best technique is long haul conduct change joined with political and natural impact, focused on expanded physical movement and some type of cognizant command over what we eat. It is anything but a convenient solution, yet it will work.

A diet that underlines dull chocolate, red wine, kale, berries, and espresso? It either seems like the most ideal street to wellbeing and weight loss, or unrealistic. However, pause, it shows signs of improvement: According to the makers of the Sirtfood Diet, these and other supposed "sirtfoods" are indicated to enact the components constrained by your body's characteristic "thin qualities" to assist you with consuming fat and get fitter.

Bragging rundown flavorful nourishment, you presumably as of now love, and supported by reports that Adele utilized it to get in shape in the wake of having a child, the Sirtfood Diet sounds naturally engaging.

Be that as it may, you don't have to destroy the chocolate and red wine high here, but science doesn't reinforce the most important dietary cases, which isn't to say that eating sirtfoods is an ill-conceived notion... Yet, similarly, as with all diets that sound unrealistic, you should take a gander at this one with a genuine examination. This is what you have to think about what sirtfoods can and can't accomplish for you.

The sirtfood eating regimen has levels that last a total of 3 weeks, after that, you can preserve "sirtifying" your food plan by means of inclusive of as many sirtfoods as possible for your meals.

The particular recipes for those two stages are observed inside the sirtfood weight loss program e-book, which was written via the weight-reduction plan's creators. You'll want to purchase it to follow the weight-reduction plan.

Most of the substances and sirtfoods are smooth to find.

But, 3 of the signature components required for those phases, Matcha inexperienced tea powder, lovage, and buckwheat, can be high priced or tough to discover.

After the Weight Loss Plan

You could repeat these two phases as regularly as favored for further weight reduction.

But I will encourage you to continue "sirtifying" with this book's guidance when you have finished those stages as you cooperate with sirtifying continuously in your daily meal.

There are a variety of sirtfood weight loss program books that are complete with recipes wealthy in sirtfoods. You may additionally consist of sirtfoods to your weight-reduction plan as a snack or in recipes you already use.

Moreover, you are advocated to maintain consuming the inexperienced juice every day.

In this way, the sirtfood weight loss plan will become greater of a lifestyle change than a one-time food regimen.

Sirtuins and Muscle Mass

There is a family of genes within the body that act as guardians of our muscle and halt its breakdown when under stress: the sirtuins. SIRT1 may be a potent inhibitor of muscle breakdown. As long as SIRT1 is activated, even once we are fasting, muscle breakdown is prevented, and that we still burn fat for fuel.

But the advantages of SIRT1 don't end with preserving muscle mass. Sirtuins actually work to extend our striated muscle mass. To elucidate how this phenomenon works, we'd like to venture into the exciting world of stem cells. Our muscle contains a special sort of somatic cell, called a satellite cell, which controls its growth and regeneration. Satellite cells just sit there quietly most of the time, but they're activated when a muscle gets damaged or stressed. This is often how our muscles get bigger through activities like weight training. SIRT1 is important for activating satellite cells, and without its activity, the muscles are significantly smaller because they do not have the capacity to develop or regenerate properly. However, by increasing SIRT1 activity, we provide a boost to our satellite cells, which inspires muscle growth and recovery.

Chapter 6: The Scientific Studies Behind the Sirt Diet

What makes the Sirtfood Diet so powerful is its ability to modify an ancient family of genes that exist in each folk. The name for this family of genes is sirtuin. So profound is that the effect of sirtuins that they're now mentioned as "master metabolic regulators." In essence, exactly what anyone eager to shed some pounds and live an extended and healthy life would want to be responsible for, which brings us nicely to fasting.

The lifelong restriction of food intake has consistently been shown to increase the anticipation of lower organisms and mammals. This remarkable finding is that the basis for the practice of caloric restriction among some people, where daily calorie intake is reduced by about 20 to 30 percent, also as its popularized offshoot, intermittent fasting, which has become a successful weight-loss diet, made famous by the likes of the 5:2 diet, or Fast Diet. While we still await proof of increased lifetime for humans from these practices, there's proof of advantages for what we'd term "healthspan"—chronic diseases drop, and fat starts to melt away.

It's not just caloric restriction and fasting that activate sirtuins; exercise does too. A bit like in fasting, sirtuins orchestrate the profound benefits of exercise. But while we are encouraged to interact in regular moderate exercise for its multitude of advantages, it's not the means through which we are meant to focus our weight-loss efforts. Research shows that the physical body has evolved ways to natural y adjust and reduce the quantity of energy we expend once we exercise, meaning that so as for exercise to be an efficient weight-loss intervention, we'd like to commit substantial time and strenuous effort. That grueling exercise regimens are the way nature intended us to take care of a healthy weight is even more dubious in light of research now suggesting that an excessive amount of exercise is often harmful, weakening our immune systems, damaging the guts, and contributing to an early death.

The main scientific evidence supporting this diet was the discovery that sirtfoods are found in the diet of people with the lowest incidence of disease and obesity rates in the world, such as the American Kuna Indians or the Japanese of Okinawa.

However, much of the weight lost comes, not exactly from the food eaten, but from the drastic cut in energy value, particularly in the first phase. Due to the restriction and the juice-based diet, the loss of water and even loss of muscle mass causes the values on the scale to decrease substantially.

In addition, the studies were carried out in people whose physical activity is high, an activity that, in itself, activates the "lean genes" and contributes to the increase in longevity.

The traditional Mediterranean diet is the one that brings together the most consensus for weight loss and health improvement, being a dietary pattern that includes several sirtfoods, such as virgin olive oil or red wine, fruit, vegetables, among others that contain vitamins and antioxidants.

It is useful to know the sirtfoods that activate sirtuin since they are healthy foods and rich in antioxidants, which enhance health and can stimulate basal metabolism.

However, the majority of weight loss will be derived from the promoted energy restriction, which is the main factor for weight loss in any diet.

The Sirtfood diet is rich in healthy foods, but not healthy eating patterns. In addition to promoting rapid weight loss without elucidating what is being lost, quite serious health claims are made without any scientific evidence to support them.

Adding SIRT-rich foods to the food day is not at all a bad idea and can bring health benefits, but this is just another restrictive diet like so many others, with nothing special worth the buzz created around it.

The sirtfood diet can't be classified as low-carb or low-fat. This diet is quite different from its many precursors while advocating many of the same things: the ingestion of fresh plant-based foods. As the name implies, this is a sirtuin based diet, but what are sirtuins, and why have you never heard about them before?

There are seven sirtuin proteins – SIRT-1 to SIRT-7. They can be found throughout your cells and the cells of every animal on the planet. Sirtuins are found in almost every living organism and in almost every part of the cell, controlling what goes on. Supplement company Elysium Health, likens the body's cells to an office with sirtuins acting as the CEO, helping the cells react to internal and external changes. They govern what is done, when it's done and who does it.

Of the seven sirtuins, one works in your cell's cytoplasm, three in the cell's mitochondria, and another three in the cell's nucleus. They have a wide number of jobs to perform, but mostly they remove acetyl groups from other proteins. These acetyl groups signal that the protein they are attached to is available to perform its function. Sirtuins remove the available flag and get the protein ready to use.

Sirtuins sound pretty crucial to your body's normal function, so why haven't you ever heard of them before?

The first sirtuin to be discovered was SIR2, a gene discovered in the 1970s which controlled the ability of fruit flies to mate. It wasn't until the 1990s that scientists discovered other similar proteins in almost every form of life. Every organism had a different number of sirtuins – bacteria has one, and yeast has five. Experiments on mice show they have the same number as humans, seven.

Sirtuins have been shown to prolong life in yeast and in mice. There is, so far, no evidence of the same effect in human beings, however, these sirtuins are present in almost every form of life, and many scientists are hopeful that if organisms as far apart as yeast and mice can see the same effect from sirtuin activation, this may also extend to humans.

In addition to sirtuins, our bodies need another substance called nicotinamide adenine dinucleotide for cells to function properly. Elysium (see above) likens this substance to the money a company needs to keep operating. Like any CEO, a sirtuin can only keep the company working properly if the cash flow is sufficient. NAD+ was first discovered in 1906. You get your supply of NAD+ from your diet by eating foods that are part of the building blocks of NAD+.

The Sirtfood Pilot Study

Bit by bit, we had pieced together all the observations from traditional cultures and findings from major scientific studies, culminating in PREDIMED, one among the simplest studies of diet ever conducted. But even the findings of PREDIMED, like many health breakthroughs, came through chance. It never began to style and test a diet of Sirtfoods. It had been only later that scientists discovered that this was effectively what PREDIMED had done.

This meant that there have been still many Sirtfoods the diet hadn't included that would have increased its immense benefits even further.

Additionally, all the research so far had established the advantages of long-term weight management and reducing disease.

But we still didn't skill quickly those benefits for weight and wellbeing might be realized. We all want to guard our future health, but don't we would like to see and feel good within the here and now too?

To answer these questions, we would have liked a purposefully conducted Sirtfood Diet intervention that included all twenty of the foremost powerful Sirtfoods that we could gather earlier measurements of the results. So, we began a pilot study of our own.

Nestled within the heart of London, England, is KX, one among Europe's most sought-after health and fitness centers. What makes KX the right place to check the consequences of the Sirtfood Diet is that it's its own restaurant, which gave us the chance not just to style the diet but to bring it to life and test it on the fitness center's members.

Our remit was clear. For seven days during a row, members would follow our carefully constructed Sirtfood Diet, and that we would meticulously track their progress from start to end, not just measuring their weight, but also monitoring changes in their body composition, which meant checking how the diet affected the amount of fat and muscle within the body. Later, we added metabolic measures to ascertain the consequences of the diet on levels of sugar (glucose) and fats (like triglycerides and cholesterol) within the blood.

The first three days were the foremost intense, with food intake restricted to 1,000 calories per day. In effect, this is often sort of a mild fast, which is vital because the lower energy intake turns down growth signals within the body and encourages it to start out clearing old debris out of cells (a process referred to as autophagy) and kick-start fat burning. But unlike popular fasting diets, this fast was mild and short-lived, making it far more sustainable, as proven by the study's exceptionally high 97.5 percent adherence rate. Plus, we wanted to research the differences that adding Sirtfoods made to the traditional downfalls experienced with fasting diets. And as we were soon to seek out, they were dramatic.

Results

The Sirtfood Diet was tested by forty and completed by thirty-nine members at KX. Of those thirty-nine, two within the trial were obese, fifteen were overweight and twenty-two had a normal/healthy body mass index (BMI). The study had a reasonably even gender split, with twenty-one women and eighteen men.

Being members of a health spa, before they started, they were more likely to exercise and remember healthy eating than the overall population.

A trick of the many diets is to use a heavily overweight and unhealthy sample of individuals to point out the advantages, as initially they reduce the quickest and most dramatically, essentially fluffing up the diet results. Our logic was the opposite: if we obtained good results with this relatively healthy group, it might set the minimum benchmark of what was achievable.

Typically, when people reduce, they're going to lose some fat, but they're going to also lose some muscle—this is par for the course when it involves dieting. We were stunned to seek out the other. Our participants either maintained their muscle or actually gained muscle. As we'll determine later within the book, this is often an infinitely more favorable sort of weight loss and a singular feature of the Sirtfood Diet.

No participant did not see improvements in body composition. And remember, all of this was achieved without dietary hardship or grueling exercise regimens.

Here's what we found:

- Participants achieved dramatic and rapid results, losing a mean of seven pounds in seven days.

- Weight loss was most noticeable around the abdominal area.

- Instead of being lost, muscle mass was either maintained or increased.

- Participants rarely felt hungry.

- Participants felt an increased sense of vitality and well -being.

- Participants reported looking better and healthier.

Chapter 7: Athletes and Famous People Who Follow the Sirt Diet

The Sirtfood Diet, also called the skinny gene-diet, is the result of the studies of the two nutritionists Aidan Goggins and Glenn Matten. Their food program, published in a volume that explains its principles and functioning, has attracted the attention of VIPs and sportsmen. Its effectiveness is based on the consumption of foods that stimulate sirtuins. As the creators of the diet of the moment explain, it is a family of genes present in each of us. They affect the ability to burn fat in addition to mood and the mechanisms that regulate longevity. It is no coincidence that they are also called "super metabolic regulators." Recent studies have shown that there are a number of foods that can stimulate sirtuins. Their consumption would, therefore, allow them to activate the metabolism and lose weight without having to undergo extreme diets.

According to nutritionists Aidan Goggins and Glen Matten, who have developed the Sirtfood Diet, the consumption of certain foods would activate sirtuins, a group of genes that stimulate the metabolism, burn fat and promote rapid weight loss.

It's one thing to urge great results following a diet during a controlled environment where all the food is expertly made and provided, and nutrition experts are available to answer any queries. It's something else altogether when people are left to defend themselves with nothing more to help them than are often found within the pages of this very book.

But it had been these reports that basically blew our minds. A diet that will so powerful y promote fat loss and improve body composition while turbocharging energy levels and well-being has many useful applications. Soon, many testimonials had poured in. From sporting superstars who were world champions and Olympic gold medalists to TV personalities and models to the most important names in showbiz, not only were they following it and sticking thereto, but they were raving about it.

Readers were smashing the 7 pounds in seven days weight loss we'd seen in our trial, proving our hypothesis we realized that it was already in shape and therefore the healthy study population was underestimating the advantages. The utmost weight loss we've seen so far was with a reporter and diet cynic who began to independently test the program's merits. Rather than bad-mouthing it, he lost 14 pounds within the first week. Safe to mention, he now joins the cohorts of converts. Faraway from the scales, others reported equally impressive results through inches lost around the waist. And better of all, the load was staying off, with the results only recuperating over the months.

Despite how fantastic all of this feedback was, for us as nutritional medicine consultants who focus on reversing and preventing disease, there was something that inspired us even more: the private stories of all the people who needed nothing more than to change their lives.

There was Robert, who had suffered depression for years. He lost 10 pounds in only a fortnight but was much more delighted with the lifting of his depressed mood, such a lot in order that he was "loving life" another time. Melanie was in terrible pain with lupus. Five weeks in, she was down 11.5 pounds, but far more important, her aches and pains had vanished. In fact, she had no lupus symptoms in the least. Feeling amazing, she not had to travel to her specialist; there was nothing to treat. And Linda, who was down a fantastic 50 pounds after three months, reversed her worsening diabetes and had the energy at another time to enjoy life again. This is often just a taste of the various inspirational stories that have are available. Heart condition has reversed. Menopause symptoms have ceased. Irritable bowel conditions have disappeared. For the primary time in years, people were sleeping well again. One perplexed ophthalmologist even contacted us with the news that after just every week on the Sirtfood Diet, her patient's chronic sclera discoloration had totally reversed and was now perfectly white again. She even sent photos for proof.

According to the studies developed by the two doctors, these genes stimulate the metabolism, cause fat burning, and promote a fairly rapid weight loss. In addition, sirtuins are able to repair cells and improve general health by transforming from slimming instruments to elixirs of longevity.

The genes of thinness, responsible for the repair and rejuvenation of cells, accelerate their activity by drawing on fat reserves and increasing resistance to diseases. The same goal can be achieved without going hungry or by eating sirtfoods. In short, fasting is of little use because the body does not receive the necessary need for nutrients and therefore triggers a series of changes in normal growth processes to survive.

The Sirtfood Diet is based on the inclusion and not on the exclusion of food, which allows you to lose more than 3 kilos in a week without undoable sacrifices. And if some of these are not so well known, most of them are known foods used in traditional cooking.

Obviously, this diet is not a magic potion, but it tries to convey how new studies help us plan a food model capable of making us lose weight by suffering less and aging in a healthy way.

Chapter 8: Over 20 Sirtfoods

When on a sirtfood diet, you have to make sure that most of the following ingredients are in your meal plan:

Arugula

Arugula is a peppery, characteristic green, which comes from the Mediterranean. It can also be called Rucola, the rocket salad, and the Italian cress. Arugula is among the Brassica or Cruciferous family. Cruciferous plants are a type of sulfur-containing dietary fibers. Glucosinolates are responsible for the bitter taste of the vegetable as well as their cancer suppression ability. Glucosinolates, including sulforaphane, are broken up into a range of beneficial compounds.

This green salad leaf (also known as Rucola) is very common in the Mediterranean diet. It is not too popular in the US food culture, and it is considered an absolute arrogance to have it on your plate. However, we're not talking about a leaf covered in gold or silver; we're talking about a green salad leaf with a peppery taste that can be used for digestive and diuretic purposes.

Buckwheat

This is one of the best sources for rutin, a sirtuin-activator nutrient. However, this crop is also amazing for ecological and sustainable farming, as it can improve the quality of the soil and prevent weed growth. However, probably the most interesting part about buckwheat is that it is a fruit seed, kind of like rhubarb, so it is not a grain at all.

There isn't a coincidence at all that buckwheat has more protein than any grain known to man, so it fits perfectly in your sirtfood diet. For every person trying to avoid gluten, this can be the ideal food. It is the ideal alternative for grains.

Capers

Some of you may not be too familiar with capers. If you haven't had the chance to taste them, you should. They are those dark-green salty things you can sometimes see on top of a pizza. Unfortunately, capers are not very used in a standard diet (it is very overlooked and underrated), but those who never had the chance to try capers don't know what they are missing. We are talking about the flower buds of the caper bush, a plant growing abundantly in the Mediterranean region. It is usually handpicked and preserved, and it has some interesting antidiabetic, anti-inflammatory, antimicrobial, antiviral, and immunomodulatory properties. Moreover, it has been used in medicine all around the Mediterranean area. Capers are also rich in sirtuin-activating nutrients, so they have the chance to shine in the sirtfood diet, and I can guarantee that you will fall in love with them.

Capers offers a cocktail of vitamins, minerals, and antioxidants with powerful anti-inflammatory effects. They contain 23 calories per 100g, and they possess large quantities of calcium, potassium, phytonutrients, vitamin K, riboflavin, iron, and copper. Quercetin and rutin have strong analgesic, antibacterial and anti-carcinogenic properties as the key antioxidants in capers. Rutin aids in the prevention and treatment of hemorrhoids, enhances circulation and reduces bad cholesterol in obese individuals. Quercetin inhibits tumor development and improves immune function. The best way to use capers is by including them in salads, pasta, and casseroles.

Celery

Celery is rich in antioxidants that help remove free radicals from your cells that promote cancer. Two anticancer compounds, apigenin and luteolin, have been identified in celery extract. Apigenin kills free radicals within the body and can promote the death of cancer cells. It also promotes autophagy. Autophagy is a mechanism in which the body destroys dysfunctional cells or components to facilitate disease prevention.

This is a plant used for thousands of years, as in ancient Egypt people were already aware of it and its properties. Back then, it was considered a medicinal plant that can be used for detoxing, cleansing and preventing diseases. Therefore, celery consumption is very good for your gut, kidney, and liver. When it was growing wildly in ancient times, it had a strong bitter flavor. However, ever since its domestication in the 17th century, celery has become a bit sweeter, and now it can be used in salads.

Chilies

This veggie should be in your diet, whether you like eating spicy food or not. It contains capsaicin, and this substance makes us savor it even more. Consuming chilies is great for activating sirtuins, and it speeds up your metabolism. In fact, the spicier the chili is, the more powerful it is when it comes to activating sirtuins. Take it easy at the beginning. You can consume Serrano peppers and then work yourself to spicier pepper. Thai chilies are very spicy, so they have a maximum sirtuin-activating effect. But to get there, you have to take it easy. Slowly work yourself to the top. When buying these peppers, make sure you select the fresh ones with deep colors. You need to avoid the soft and wrinkled ones.

Cocoa

Cocoa was considered sacred by the Aztecs and Mayans, and it was a food type reserved only for the warriors or the elite. It was often used as a currency, as people were aware of its value. Although back then it was mostly used as a drink, you don't have to dilute it with milk or water to reap the full benefits of it. The best way to consume cocoa is by eating dark chocolate (with at least 85 percent solid cocoa). However, this also depends on how the chocolate is made, as this product is usually treated with an alkalizing agent, which is known to lower the acidity of the chocolate and give it a darker color.

Coffee

This is a drink enjoyed by most adults out there, and it is considered indispensable by most of them. We even believe that we can function without a cup of coffee to start within the morning. Obviously, that's not true, but we can honestly believe that coffee significantly improves our productivity and our daily activities. Caffeine acid is a nutrient known to activate sirtuins, so there's more to drinking coffee than a popular and very pleasant social activity. Coffee houses all over the world are making serious money out of people's addiction to hanging out and drinking coffee.

Extra-Virgin Olive Oil

This oil is perhaps the healthiest form of fats you can think of, and it is not missing from any salad in the Mediterranean diet. The health benefits of consuming this oil are countless. It prevents and fights against diabetes, different types of cancer, osteoporosis, and many more. Plus, the extra-virgin olive oil can be associated with increased longevity, as it also has anti-aging effects. You can easily find this type of oil in most supermarkets, so you don't have any excuse to exclude it from your sirtfood diet. This oil has the right nutrients to activate the sirtuin gene in your body.

Garlic

As you probably know, it has an antifungal and antibiotic effect and has been successfully used to treat stomach ulcers. Plus, it can be used to remove waste products from your body. It has amazing effects on your blood pressure, blood sugar level, and heart. So why refuse this delicious food to feel healthy? Garlic contains allicin, a nutrient capable of triggering sirtuins, but this nutrient can only be valued if the garlic clove is crushed. Therefore, if you want to reap the benefits of this food, you have to avoid cooking it immediately. You need to crush it first and let the allicin form (should take around 10 minutes) before cooking it. This is the right way to use garlic in a sirtfood diet.

Green Tea

Green Tea loaded with the most important natural medicines, antioxidants, and cancer-fighting compounds. The drink consists of dried leaves from the Camellia sinensis plant, which are effective for pancreatic cancer, cancer of the prostate, lung cancer, and colorectal cancer. Green tea also reduces bad cholesterol, reduces the risk of heart disease, and protects from a stroke. Science supports its weight loss benefits. Green tea is rich in polyphenols that reduce inflammation and contribute to cancer control.

In some cultures, drinking tea is as popular as drinking coffee, but what if you find the tea assortment that works best for you? It is true that you can have tea from various medicinal plants, and they all have positive effects on your health. However, most of these plants are focused on preventing or fighting a specific disease. Have you ever thought about drinking tea for your wellbeing or to feel great? Well, this is what green tea is for. First appeared in Asia, green tea has become very popular in Western culture. It has plenty of antioxidants. It can be used for detox, and it speeds up your metabolism. But there's a lot more to drinking green tea than these. Its benefits expand to preventing and fighting against diabetes, heart diseases, and cancer in incipient forms. When it comes to sirtuins activation, green tea contains EGCG (epigallocatechin), which is known to be a very powerful sirtuin activator.

Kale

Kale is very rich in nutrients with very low calories, which makes it one of the world's most nutrient-dense foods. Several strong antioxidants such as Quercetin and Kaempferol are found in kale, and they have numerous positive health effects. Kale contains vitamin C, an antioxidant with several important roles in the body. Kale contains bile acid-binding substances that lower the levels of cholesterol. Throughout test tube and animal studies, Kale contains compounds that have been shown to help combat cancer; however, human evidence is still conflicting.

You can never go wrong with some leafy greens, and this is applicable for kale as well. Perhaps not many of you have tried it before, but it is totally worth it. Over the last few years, kale has gained a lot of popularity and appreciation from both nutritionists and consumers, and they have all the reasons to like and appreciate it. But what's all the fuss about it? How come this vegetable has become so popular lately? We can go on for hours talking about the health benefits of kale, but let's stick to the ones relevant to sirtuins, shall we? This leafy green is one of the best sources of kaempferol and quercetin, nutrients capable of triggering sirtuins. Therefore, kale should not be missing from your sirtfood diet, and you can easily make your own juices using it. Another great fact about kale is that it is not something exotic, a very rare vegetable available on a remote tropical island. This leafy green can be grown locally, so it is very accessible and affordable.

Medjool Dates

If you have the chance to go to any country in the Middle East or the Arabian Peninsula, you will find that dates are a very common snack. Dehydrated, covered in chocolate, or in a fresher form, dates are perhaps the most common snack you can find over there. Now you are probably wondering if it has any health benefits, especially if you find out that Medjool dates have around 66 percent sugar. But sugar in this form is a lot less harmful than processed or refined sugar, which doesn't have any sirtuin-activating properties and can be easily linked to weight gain (even obesity), heart disease, and diabetes.

Parsley

The parsley leaves are extremely frequent in recipes, so it is not missing from the sirtfood diet. You can chop them and toss them in your meal or use a sprig for decorative purposes. But parsley is not for decorating your plate, as you are not trying to impress a jury of famous chefs. This is an underrated plant. In ancient times, parsley was eaten after a meal to refresh the breath, so it was not considered as part of a meal. The sirtfood diet puts parsley where it belongs, and that is on your plate as an important part of your meal. With its refreshing and vibrant taste, parsley finally receives the respect it deserves.

Red Endive

This vegetable is one of the latest discoveries in the world of plants. How come? It was discovered by accident in 1830 when a Belgian farmer who stored chicory roots in his cellar forgot about them and discovered them with white leaves that happened to be crunchy, tender, and delicious. The recently found plant is growing all over the world and plays a major role in a sirtfood diet because of its high concentration of luteolin, a sirtuin-activating nutrient. On top of that, luteolin has been used to improve sociability for autistic children. Judging, by the way, most of us raise our kids (isolated, just with technology), more and more kids tend to be autistic. Therefore, the red endive can be very helpful in this case, so you better include it on your shopping list.

Red Onions

If you are only eating onions as O-rings with your burger, then you better rethink the way you consume this incredible vegetable. This type of onion has a sweeter taste (compared to yellow onion). It has plenty of antioxidants, and it is known to fight against inflammation, heart diseases, and diabetes. But there's a lot more to the red onion than meets the eye. It is a great source for quercetin, an amazing sirtuin-activating nutrient that is believed to enhance sports performance. Therefore, the red onion is a must in your sirtfood diet.

Red Wine

Red wine is made when dark-colored, whole grapes are fermented. It has high antioxidants effects. Moderate intake of the drink is good for health. The potent compounds in red wine have been associated with many health benefits, like reduced inflammation, lower risk of cancer and heart disease, and longevity. Taking 1–2 glasses of red wine every day can reduce the risk of heart and stroke disease. High amounts can, however, increase the risk. Moderate consumption of red wine can reduce the risk of multiple cancers, dementia, and depression. It can also improve insulin sensitivity and decrease women's risk of developing type 2 diabetes.

The Mediterranean diet encourages the consumption of red wine, and there are plenty of reasons why you should consider moderate consumption of it. We are not going to talk about the effects it has on your blood, blood sugar level, and so on. Not even about how moderate consumption can decrease the death rates by heart disease. Or about how red wine can prevent common colds and cavities (yes, it can even improve your oral health). Red wines like Merlot, Cabernet Sauvignon, or Pinot Noir have an incredible concentration of polyphenol to activate your sirtuins. Again, moderate consumption is essential, so one glass of wine should be more than enough.

Soy

There is a whole food-processing industry behind soy, as it is used to create food products for vegetarians. But let's face it — drinking soymilk will not activate your sirtuins. Industrially processed food is not very recommended for your health, so it should be excluded from your sirtfood diet. In natural form, soy contains formononetin and daidzein, two great sirtuin-activating nutrients. For this kind of diet, you need to consider soy in different forms. Consider tofu (the vegan protein boost) or different fermented forms of soy, such as natto, tempeh, or miso (a Japanese fermented paste with an intense umami flavor).

Strawberries

Of all the fruits out there, strawberries are among the ones with the most health benefits. Yes, they are sweet, but they happen to have a very high concentration of fisetin, a nutrient that can activate sirtuins. What is very confusing is that strawberries are known to prevent heart diseases, diabetes, cancer, osteoporosis, and Alzheimer's disease. They are even associated with healthy aging. Although they are sweet, 3½ ounces of strawberries only contain a teaspoon of sugar.

The consumption of this fruit can lower the insulin demand, basically turning the food into a sustainable energy releaser. There is research claiming that eating strawberries has similar effects on drug therapy for a person suffering from diabetes.

Turmeric

You are probably familiar with the effects ginger has on your overall health, but you don't know what turmeric can do for you. This plant is related to ginger, and it is very appreciated throughout Asia for medical and culinary reasons. India is responsible for 80 percent of the whole turmeric on the planet, and some nutritionists refer to it as the "golden spice" or "India's gold." Why is that? Because it contains curcumin, a very rare sirtuin-activating nutrient. Unfortunately, this nutrient is very poorly assimilated when eaten, but if you cook it in liquid, add some fat and black pepper, you can boost its absorption. It is no wonder that turmeric fits so well in traditional Indian cuisine, as it goes very well with black pepper and ghee in hot dishes or curries.

Turmeric is a substance that contains strong anti-inflammatory and antioxidant characteristics, curcumin. Most studies used turmeric extracts that include standard quantities of curcumin. Curcumin suppresses many molecules that play major roles in inflammation. The effects of curcumin are potent. It neutralizes free radicals and stimulates the antioxidant enzymes of the body. Curcumin boosts brain hormone BDNF levels that increase neuronal growth and combat various degenerative processes in your brain. This natural compound, Curcumin, reduces body inflammation to avoid arthritis, chronic pain, cancer, cardiovascular disease, and numerous degenerative conditions. Turmeric also improves the capacity of the body to provide an antioxidant effect, prevents radial damage, and improves brain function. It contains BDNF (brain-derived neurotrophic factor), a protein that helps nerve cells to grow, mature, and survive.

Walnuts

Walnuts are a great source of antioxidants that can help to combat atherosclerosis, a type of oxidative damages in your body, including damages resulting from bad LDL cholesterol. They are an excellent source of plant omega-3 fat that can contribute to reducing the risk of heart disease. Several components and nutrients in walnuts may contribute to a reduction of inflammation, which in many chronic conditions is the main culprit. Walnuts are not only beneficial to you, but they also nourish the good bacteria residing in your intestine.

As it happens, the walnut tree is the oldest food tree known to humans, as it was discovered around 7,000 BCE. Its original location was in ancient Persia (modern-day Iran), and now this tree is spread all around the world, as it can easily adapt to different climates of the globe. In the United States, walnuts are a success story. California is the biggest producer of walnuts in the United States, responsible for 99 percent of the US commercial supply and for three-quarters of the walnut trade worldwide. Without any doubt, walnuts are the best nuts when it comes to health.

Dark Chocolate

Dark chocolate has minerals like iron, magnesium, and zinc. Its content of cocoa possesses antioxidants known as flavonoids, which have numerous health benefits. Chocolate is made out of cacao, a plant with an elevated level of minerals and antioxidants. Dark chocolate contains much higher amounts of cacao with reducing sugar than commercial milk chocolate. Dark chocolate contains polyphenols and flavanols that have antioxidant properties. Antioxidants are substances that neutralize free radicals, thereby preventing oxidative stress. Oxidative stress results from the excessive circulation of free radicals and contributes to the natural aging process. Oxidative stress can also contribute to a range of diseases, such as Parkinson's, heart disease, diabetes, Alzheimer's disease, eye disease, and cancer.

Blueberries

The blueberry is rich in vitamin C, vitamin K, copper, manganese, and dietary fibers. Their antioxidant content is also the highest in all berries. These popular Sirtfoods improve immunity and neutralize free radicals, which can harm the structure of the cells. They are ideal for dieters who want low calories and carbohydrates. Recent studies indicate that blueberries can reduce stomach fat and risk factors that lead to metabolic syndrome. They are high in calcium; therefore, improve bone health and prevent osteoporosis.

Tofu

Tofu contains all nine essential amino acids, which is a good protein source. This plant is also a precious source of iron, calcium, manganese, phosphorous, magnesium, copper, zinc, and vitamin B1. It is believed that soy protein where tofu is produced helps to improve bad cholesterol (LDL) levels. It brings relief to some symptoms of menopause.

Chapter 9: Top Tips for Sirt Dieting

Fat burning, increasing muscles, and better cellular fitness—these are the guaranteed results of the SirtFood diet.

Being healthy and losing weight is an everyday choice. You have to take those first baby steps and see how it can change you and your life.

If you want to reap the amazing results of SirtFoods, here are some suggested ways to jumpstart your diet:

Safety first - Before starting any particular diet or regimen, consult your healthcare provider, especially if you have an existing illness. This will ensure that the diet will not sabotage any medications that you might be taking or have an adverse effect on your health. Do not worry, the SirtFood diet is fairly safe.

Knowledge is power - This diet is still brand new, but there is still a good amount of information available and more upcoming since this diet is fast gaining popularity. In addition, you can also search the internet for recipes, food alternatives, nutrient content, and more.

Follow the guidelines - SirtFood is guaranteed to bring results, if and only if you carefully follow the diet guide and suggested food.

Help yourself - Aside from following what is allowed in the food program, you can start by eliminating processed and starchy food from your normal diet. Stop eating junk! This will fast track the result of the SirtFood Diet.

Start a physical activity - SirtFood diet can indeed burn those fats and build muscle, but I recommend that you start adding physical activities to your daily routine. A 30-minute walk a day would do wonders for your body and will also fast track the results. In addition, there are many wonderful effects when exercising like preventing and combating health conditions, helping improve your mood, promoting better sleep, burning calories, giving you an energy boost, and more.

Hit the supermarket - The SirtFood diet depends on certain foods. These foods were chosen because of their sirtuin-triggering ability. So if you do not follow the list, well, you won't see results. Do not worry, because I will be providing a list of suggested foods; Plus, there are no overly expensive types of foods, and you can find them readily available almost anywhere (you might even already have some lurking in your fridge).

Be ready with the initial "restrictions" - Of course, if you want to see different results, you have to "sacrifice" a little in order to achieve the full benefits of the SirtFood diet. But don't worry, the first three days are only the hardest ones for this diet since there will be calorie restrictions involved, but rest assured that it will become easier each day. Although for others who tried the diet, the restrictions set was not that hard for them, the reason is careful planning of meals. You will not go hungry with this diet if you choose wisely.

Plan your meals ahead - Whatever diet you may be on, planning your meals is a big help. Not only will it reduce the stress from dieting, but you can also have the chance to weigh your choices and fill in your cupboard. For the first phase of this diet (I will be elaborating that in Chapter 4), you have to follow a calorie count. You will be surprised that there are many filling dishes allowed with fewer calories and packed with sirtuins.

Involve a diet partner - This diet could also greatly benefit your family, partner, or friends (not only for overweight individuals), plus it is easier when you have an accountability partner to remind you, share recipes with or even cook dishes with.

Document your progress - You can start by taking "before" pictures and take necessary body measurements. You could also keep a food diary so that you can watch your food intake. Observe the changes in your body with each week or phase. You can also have a set of goals to further push you to continue with the diet.

Be kind to yourself - Do not set too high expectations. Yes, some can easily lose 7 pounds in a week, but remember that our bodies are not all the same; and of course, your level of commitment will also count. Other variables could be adding an exercise regimen to the diet plan, which could make the losing weight process faster.

Chapter 10: Shopping for the Sirt Diet

When compiling your shopping list, make sure you rule any sort of processed food and the most potent source of carbs. Forget about chips, doughnuts, and other forms of processed sweets or salty snacks. You need to replace them with healthy fruits like walnuts, strawberries, blueberries, dates, and other fruits or seeds. Your desserts or snacks don't have to be tasteless; they can be, in fact, extremely delicious. Who doesn't like eating strawberries, blueberries, or even walnuts?

Another thing you need to consider is to rule out any soda and most juices. Why? Because they contain too much sugar, and too much sugar is extremely harmful to your body. You will have the chance to drink a lot of green healthy juices and some other drinks rich in sirtuins, like coffee, cocoa, green tea, and red wine (but moderately). A good drink can be milk with cocoa, but instead of regular skimmed, semi-skimmed, or whole milk, you can just go for the soy milk.

It is true that sirtuins can be found mostly in fruits and vegetables, but this doesn't mean you have to become a vegetarian in order to eat sirtfoods. Therefore, your shopping list can include meat or fish as well. You can use sirtfoods as a garnish or as condiments, but you also need to realize that you don't buy fruits and vegetables just for their antioxidants and vitamins. They have a lot more value to you, as they represent minor stress to your cells, similar to exercise and fasting.

However, when buying products, you need to buy less (in quantity) and more often. There is no need to stock them in your home, as they are very perishable. Plus, you need them as fresh as possible, so it is better to buy them from a grocery store if you know they are always bringing in fresh produce.

This book will provide you detailed recipes and even a meal plan you can follow, so all the ingredients you need can be found in the recipes. Follow these recipes strictly, and you will quickly notice how you can lose plenty of pounds starting from your first week of the meal plan.

To recap, when doing your shopping, you need to remember the following:

- Rule out processed food and replace it with sirtfood when possible (check the top 20 sirtfoods from the previous chapter).

- Stay away from any sweets or snacks with a very high calorie and carb intake. Snacks are where you can make a difference, as you can eat sirtfood snacks like walnuts, strawberries, and blueberries.

- Don't bother buying sodas or juices. You will have the opportunity to create your own green healthy juices.

- Make sure you include in your shopping list strawberries, blueberries, walnuts, and other fruits or seeds.

- Buy coffee, green tea, cocoa, and red wine (in smaller quantities).

- Your shopping list should not consist just of the 20 ingredients and foods mentioned in the previous chapter, so you don't have to become a vegetarian (meat is allowed as well).

- If you are using meat, make sure you use sirtfoods to garnish it or spice the meat.

Chapter 11: Complete Four-Week Plan

Let's be frank right from the beginning! You simply can't lose weight and boost your health overnight — this can only happen in time. The sirtfood diet is not a collection of recipes for magic potions. Although we encourage you to make the sirtfood diet your default meal plan, the best way to find out if a diet is working is to monitor your results. In terms of weight loss, this can be so easily done, as you can check your weight on the scale on a daily basis (more sophisticated scales can even show your BMI), measure yourself around the waist, or check yourself in the mirror to notice any visible results. Obviously, medical results can't be monitored on a daily basis, as health improvements can only happen in time. If you have the right equipment, you can measure your blood pressure and tools on a daily basis. There are plenty of health apps you can install on your smartphone to monitor different health indicators.

Therefore, you need a minimum period of time to test the sirtfood diet, and the optimum time is four weeks. This period should be more than enough to show you the first signs of improvement when it comes to your health. So feel free to run a blood analysis after these four weeks and monitor the triglyceride, cholesterol, and blood sugar level. There are a lot of indicators you can get from blood analysis, but there is no better proof that this diet really works.

This program requires preparation to make the transition from your default diet to the sirtfood one. Plenty of people are very stressed and just want to lose a lot of weight by constraining themselves to eat just a few ingredients. The sirtfood diet is not like that, and it encourages you to try all sorts of ingredients. However, it helps you to combine them in such a way that reaps most of the weight loss and health benefits. The founders of this diet, Aidan Goggins and Glen Matten, like to think that this is a diet of inclusion and no food is left behind. If you check the recipes included in this book, you will see that these foods use a wide range of ingredients. You can have standard or vegan meals in order to enjoy diversity.

Sounds neat, right? You probably tried a lot of restrictive diets and perhaps even fasting. You either couldn't stick to a radical diet or had nasty side effects after following (it was not good for your health, or you started to gain weight immediately after quitting it). Perhaps you are simply not satisfied with the results. This is where the sirtfood diet can help you. So why not lose weight in a healthy and sustainable way? The cure to our medical problems caused by bad nutrition can be this interesting diet. Since this diet is very recent, perhaps you don't know anyone who has tried it before. Wouldn't it be great if you had the opportunity to test the meal plan before your friends and relatives try it? How would you feel if you were envied for your physical shape and overall health? And when somebody asks you about your secret, you can mention the sirtfood diet.

Well, this diet should deliver amazing results after just four weeks. This is why I encourage you to try for the four-week program (at least). If you are satisfied with the results (and I have a hunch you will), then it is highly recommended to stick to this diet in the long term to make it your default one. Therefore, if this diet works for you, why change it with a different one? Four weeks should be sufficient to find out whether the diet is appropriate for you or not.

This weight loss plan is based totally on studies on sirtuins (sirts), a collection of seven proteins discovered within the body that has been proven to adjust an effect of capabilities, consisting of Metabolism, irritation, and lifespan.

Certain natural plant compounds can be capable of increase the level of those proteins within the body, and meals containing them were dubbed "sirtfoods."

The eating regimen's creators declare that following the sirtfood weight loss program will cause speedy weight reduction, all while retaining muscle mass and shielding you from chronic Ailments.

Once you are done with the diet, you're recommended to retain which include sirtfoods and the diet's signature inexperienced juice into your ordinary weight loss plan.

Chapter 12: Breakfast

Strawberry & Citrus Blend

Preparation time: 30 min

Cooking time: 0 min

Servings: 1

Ingredients:

- 75g (3oz) strawberries

- 1 apple, cored

- 1 orange, peeled

- ½ avocado, peeled and de-stoned

- ½ teaspoon matcha powder

- Juice of 1 lime

Directions:

1. Place all of the ingredients into a blender with enough water to cover them and process until smooth.

Grapefruit & Celery Blast

Preparation time: 30 min

Cooking time: 0 min

Servings: 1

Ingredients:

- 1 grapefruit, peeled

- 2 stalks of celery

- 50g (2oz) kale

- ½ teaspoon matcha powder

Directions:

1. Place all the ingredients into a blender with enough water to cover them and blitz until smooth.

Orange & Celery Crush

Preparation time: 30 min

Cooking time: 0 min

Servings: 1

Ingredients:

- 1 carrot, peeled

- 3 stalks of celery

- 1 orange, peeled

- ½ teaspoon matcha powder

- Juice of 1 lime

Directions:

1. Place all of the ingredients into a blender with enough water to cover them and blitz until smooth.

Tropical Chocolate Delight

Preparation time: 30 min

Cooking time: 0 min

Servings: 1

Ingredients:

- 1 mango, peeled & de-stoned

- 75g (3oz) fresh pineapple, chopped

- 50g (2oz) kale

- 25g (1oz) rocket

- 1 tablespoon 100% cocoa powder or cacao nibs

- 150mls (5fl oz) coconut milk

Directions:

1. Place all of the ingredients into a blender and blitz until smooth. You can add a little water if it seems too thick.

Walnut & Spiced Apple Tonic

Preparation time: 30 min

Cooking time: 0 min

Servings: 1

Ingredients:

- 6 walnuts halves

- 1 apple, cored

- 1 banana

- ½ teaspoon matcha powder

- ½ teaspoon cinnamon

- Pinch of ground nutmeg

Directions:

1. Place all of the ingredients into a blender and add sufficient water to cover them. Blitz until smooth and creamy.

Pineapple & Cucumber Smoothie

Preparation time: 30 min

Cooking time: 0 min

Servings: 1

Ingredients:

- 50g (2oz) cucumber

- 1 stalk of celery

- 2 slices of fresh pineapple

- 2 sprigs of parsley

- ½ teaspoon matcha powder

- A squeeze of lemon juice

Directions:

1. Place all of the ingredients into a blender with enough water to cover them and blitz until smooth.

Sweet Rocket (Arugula) Boost

Preparation time: 30 min

Cooking time: 0 min

Servings: 1

Ingredients:

- 25g (1oz) fresh rocket (arugula) leaves

- 75g (3oz) kale

- 1 apple

- 1 carrot

- 1 tablespoon fresh parsley

- Juice of 1 lime

Directions:

1. Place all of the ingredients into a blender with enough water to cover and process until smooth.

Sirtfood Mushroom Scrambled Eggs

Preparation time: 10 min

Cooking time: 20 min

Servings: 1

Ingredients:

- 1 teaspoon ground garlic

- 1 carrot

- Eggs

- 1 teaspoon mild curry powder

- 20g lettuce, approximately sliced

- 1 teaspoon extra virgin olive oil

- A couple of mushrooms, finely chopped

- 5g parsley, finely chopped

- Optional - insert a seed mix for a topper plus some rooster sauce for taste

Directions:

1. Mix the curry and garlic powder, and then add just a little water until you've achieved a light glue.

2. Steam the lettuce for 2 - 3 minutes.

3. Heat the oil in a skillet over moderate heat and fry the chili and mushrooms 2-3 minutes until they've begun to soften and brown.

4. Insert the eggs and spice paste and cook over moderate heat, then add the carrot and then proceed to cook over moderate heat for a further minute. In the end, put in the parsley, mix well and serve.

Blue Hawaii Smoothie

Preparation time: 10 min

Cooking time: 20 min

Servings: 1

Ingredients:

- ½ cup frozen tomatoes

- Two tbsp ground flaxseed

- ⅛ cup tender coconut (unsweetened, organic)

- Few walnuts

- ½ cup fat-free yogurt

- 5-6 ice cubes

- Splash of water

Directions:

1. Throw all of the ingredients together and combine until smooth. You might need to shake it or put more water in the mix.

Turkey Breakfast Sausages

Preparation time: 5 Minutes

Cooking time: 55 Minutes

Servings: 2

Ingredients:

- 1 lb extra lean ground turkey

- 1 tbsp (EVOO 9 Extra Virgin Olive Oil) and a little more to coat the pan

- 1 tbsp fennel seeds

- 2 teaspoons smoked paprika

- 1 teaspoon red pepper flakes

- 1 teaspoon peppermint

- 1 teaspoon chicken seasoning

- A couple of shredded cheddar cheese

- A couple of chives, finely chopped

- A few shakes of garlic and onion powder

- Two spins of pepper and salt

Directions:

1. Preheat oven to 350 F.

2. Utilize a little EVOO to grease a miniature muffin pan.

3. Combine all ingredients and blend thoroughly.

4. Fill each pit on top of the pan and then cook for approximately 15-20 minutes. Each toaster differs, therefore when muffin temperature is 165°, remove.

Chapter 13: Quick Fixes

Honey Mustard Dressing

Preparation time: 10 minutes

Cooking time: 0 minutes

Servings: 2

Ingredients:

- 4 tablespoon Olive oil

- 1 ½ teaspoon Honey

- 1 ½ teaspoon Mustard

- 1 teaspoon Lemon juice

- 1 pinch Salt

Directions:

1. Mix olive oil, honey, mustard, and lemon juice into an even dressing with a whisk.

2. Season with salt.

Amazing Garlic Aioli

Preparation time: 5 minutes

Cooking time: 0 minutes

Servings: 3

Ingredients:

- ½ cup mayonnaise, low fat and low sodium

- 2 garlic cloves, minced

- Juice of 1 lemon

- 1 tablespoon fresh-flat leaf Italian parsley, chopped

- 1 teaspoon chives, chopped

- Salt and pepper to taste

Directions:

1. Add mayonnaise, garlic, parsley, lemon juice, chives, and season with salt and pepper.

2. Blend until combined well.

3. Pour into refrigerator and chill for 30 minutes.

4. Serve and use as needed!

Paleo Chocolate Wraps with Fruits

Preparation time: 25 minutes

Cooking time: 0 minutes

Servings: 2

Ingredients:

- 4 pieces Egg

- 100 ml Almond milk

- 2 tablespoons Arrowroot powder

- 4 tablespoons Chestnut flour

- 1 tablespoon Olive oil (mild)

- 2 tablespoons Maple syrup

- 2 tablespoons Cocoa powder

- 1 tablespoon Coconut oil

- 1 piece Banana

- 2 pieces Kiwi (green)

- 2 pieces Mandarins

Directions:

1. Mix all ingredients (except fruit and coconut oil) into an even dough.

2. Melt some coconut oil in a small pan and pour a quarter of the batter into it.

3. Bake it like a pancake baked on both sides.

4. Place the fruit in a wrap and serve it lukewarm.

5. A wonderfully sweet start to the day!

Vegetarian Curry from the Crock Pot

Preparation time: 6 hours 10 minutes

Cooking time: 6 hours

Servings: 2

Ingredients:

- 4 pieces Carrot

- 2 pieces Sweet potato

- 1 piece Onion

- 3 cloves Garlic

- 2 tablespoon Curry powder

- 1 teaspoon Ground caraway (ground)

- ¼ teaspoon Chili powder

- ¼ teaspoon Celtic sea salt

- 1 pinch Cinnamon

- 100 ml vegetable broth

- 400 g Tomato cubes (can)

- 250 g Sweet peas

- 2 tablespoon tapioca flour

Directions:

1. Roughly chop vegetables and potatoes and press garlic. Halve the sugar snap peas.

2. Put the carrots, sweet potatoes, and onions in the slow cooker.

3. Mix tapioca flour with curry powder, cumin, chili powder, salt, and cinnamon, and sprinkle this mixture on the vegetables.

4. Pour the vegetable broth over it.

5. Close the lid of the slow cooker and let it simmer for 6 hours on a low setting.

6. Stir in the tomatoes and sugar snap peas for the last hour.

7. Cauliflower rice is a great addition to this dish.

Chapter 14: Lunch

Greek Sea Bass Mix

Preparation time: 10 minutes

Cooking time: 22 minutes

Servings: 2

Ingredients:

- 2 sea bass fillets, boneless
- 1 garlic clove, minced
- 5 cherry tomatoes, halved
- 1 tablespoon chopped parsley
- 2 shallots, chopped
- Juice of ½ lemon
- 1 tablespoon olive oil
- 8 ounces baby spinach
- Cooking spray

Directions:

1. Grease a baking dish with cooking oil, then add the fish, tomatoes, parsley, and garlic. Drizzle the lemon juice over the fish, cover the dish and place it in the oven at 350 degrees F.

2. Bake for 15 minutes and then divide between plates. Heat up a pan with the olive oil over medium heat, add shallot, stir and cook for 1 minute. Add spinach, stir, cook for 5 minutes more, add to the plate with the fish and serve.

3. Enjoy!

Pomegranate Guacamole

Preparation time: 10 Minutes

Cooking time: 40 Minutes

Servings: 4

Ingredients:

- The flesh of 2 ripe avocados

- Seeds from 1 pomegranate

- 1 bird's-eye chili pepper, finely chopped

- ½ red onion, finely chopped

- Juice of 1 lime

Directions:

1. Place the avocado, onion, chili, and lime juice into a blender and process until smooth. Stir in the pomegranate seeds. Chill before serving. Serve as a dip for chop vegetables.

Chicken Curry with Potatoes and Kale

Preparation time: 10 Minutes

Cooking time: 20 Minutes

Servings: 4

Ingredients:

- 600g chicken breast, cut into pieces

- 4 tablespoons of extra virgin olive oil

- 3 tablespoons turmeric

- 2 red onions, sliced

- 2 red chilies, finely chopped

- 3 cloves of garlic, finely chopped

- 1 tablespoon freshly chopped ginger

- 1 tablespoon curry powder

- 1 tin of small tomatoes (400ml)

- 500ml chicken broth

- 200ml coconut milk

- 2 pieces cardamom

- 1 cinnamon stick

- 600g potatoes mainly waxy

- 10g parsley, chopped

- 175g kale, chopped

- 5g coriander, chopped

Directions:

1. Marinate the chicken in a teaspoon of olive oil and a tablespoon of turmeric for about 30 minutes. Then fry in a high frying pan at high heat for about 4 minutes. Remove from the pan and set aside.

2. Heat a tablespoon of oil in a pan with chili, garlic, onion, and ginger. Boil everything over medium heat and then add the curry powder and a tablespoon of turmeric and cook for another two minutes, stirring occasionally. Add tomatoes, cook for another two minutes until finally chicken stock, coconut milk, cardamom, and cinnamon stick are added. Cook for about 45 to 60 minutes and add some broth if necessary.

3. In the meantime, preheat the oven to 425 °. Peel and chop the potatoes. Bring water to the boil, add the potatoes with turmeric and cook for 5 minutes. Then pour off the water and let it evaporate for about 10 minutes. Spread olive oil together with the potatoes on a baking tray and bake in the oven for 30 minutes.

4. When the potatoes and curry are almost ready, add the coriander, kale, and chicken and cook for five minutes until the chicken is hot.

5. Add parsley to the potatoes and serve with the chicken curry.

Mushroom & Tofu Scramble

Preparation time: 30 minutes

Cooking time: 15 minutes

Servings: 1

Ingredients:

- 100g tofu, extra firm

- 1 tsp ground turmeric

- 1 tsp extra virgin olive oil

- 20g red onion, thinly sliced

Directions:

1. Place 2 sheets of kitchen towel under and on top of the tofu, then rest a considerable weight such as saucepan onto the tofu to ensure it drains off the liquid.

2. Combine the curry powder, turmeric, and 1-2 tsp of water to form a paste. Using a steamer, cook kale for 3-4 minutes.

3. In a skillet, warm oil over medium heat. Add the chili, mushrooms, and onion, cooking for several minutes or until brown and tender.

4. Break the tofu into small pieces and toss in the skillet. Coat with the spice paste and stir, ensuring everything becomes evenly coated. Cook for up to 5 minutes, or until the tofu has browned, then add the kale and fry for 2 more minutes. Garnish with parsley before serving.

Chapter 15: Super Salads

Coronation Chicken Salad

Preparation time: 10 minutes

Cooking time: 45 minutes

Servings: 2

Ingredients:

- 75 g Natural yogurt

- Juice of ¼ of a lemon

- 1 tsp Coriander, hacked

- 1 tsp ground turmeric

- 1/2 tsp Mild curry powder

- 100 g Cooked chicken bosom, cut into scaled-down pieces

- 6 Walnut parts, finely hacked

- 1 Medjool date, finely hacked

- 20 g Red onion, diced

- 1 Birds eye stew

- 40 g Rocket to serve

Directions:

1. Blend the yogurt, lemon juice, coriander, and flavors together in a bowl. Include all the rest of the fixings and serve on a bed of the rocket.

Spring Salad with Strawberry Vinaigrette

Preparation time: 10 minutes

Cooking time: 50 minutes

Servings: 3

Ingredients:

- 2 cups Kale, curly, chopped

- 1 cup Red cabbage, shredded

- 1 cup Arugula

- 1 Carrot, grated

- ½ Red onion, finely sliced

- 1 rib Celery, finely chopped

- ½ cup Parsley, chopped –

- ½ cup Walnuts, toasted and chopped

- ½ cup Blueberries

- 1 Boiled egg, sliced

- ¼ cup Blue cheese or feta cheese, crumbled

- ¼ cup Chicken breast, cooked, diced

- ¼ cup Strawberries, frozen

- ¼ teaspoon Black pepper, ground

- 1 tablespoon Extra virgin olive oil

- 1 tablespoon Apple cider vinegar

- 1 Medjool dates, pitted

- ½ teaspoon Sea salt

Directions:

1. Begin by making the strawberry vinaigrette. To do this, add the frozen strawberries, black pepper, olive oil, apple cider vinegar, Medjool date, and sea salt all into a blender. Blend on high until the vinaigrette is completely smooth with no clumps. Set aside.

2. Add the vegetables, blueberries, walnuts, and parsley to a bowl together, and toss them to combine. Drizzle the prepared vinaigrette over the salad and then toss again.

3. Over the top of your salad sprinkle the boiled egg, cheese, and chicken. Divide out the servings and enjoy immediately. If you wish to prepare your salad ahead of time, hold off on adding the vinaigrette until the last moment to avoid wilting.

Rainbow Salad with Lemon Vinaigrette

Preparation time: 10 minutes

Cooking time: 60 minutes

Servings: 3

Ingredients:

- 2 cups Sweet potatoes, diced
- 2 cups Brussels sprouts, shredded
- 2 cups Red cabbage, shredded
- 3 cups Kale, chopped
- 1 cup Buckwheat groats, cooked
- 1 cup Fresh cherries, pitted and sliced
- 1 tablespoon Extra virgin olive oil
- ¼ cup Almonds, sliced
- 2 ½ tablespoons Lemon juice
- 1 teaspoon Sea salt, divided
- 2 teaspoons Date paste
- ⅓ cup Extra virgin olive oil
- ¼ teaspoon Black pepper, ground

Directions:

1. Allow your oven to heat to Fahrenheit four-hundred and twenty-five degrees while you prepare the sweet potatoes. To do this, add the sweet potatoes onto a baking sheet and toss them in a single tablespoon of olive oil and half of the sea salt.

2. Place the sweet potato cubes in the oven and allow them to roast until they are fork-tender and lightly browned, about twenty-five minutes.

3. Bring the chopped kale to a large salad bowl and massage it with your hands until it is tender. This step makes a big difference, so don't skip it! Add in the cabbage, Brussels sprouts, cherries, almonds, roasted sweet potatoes, and buckwheat groats. Toss them all together.

4. In another bowl, use a whisk and vigorously combine the remaining olive oil, date paste, black pepper, lemon juice, and the remaining sea salt. Once the vinaigrette has emulsified, pour it over your salad and toss until it is evenly coated. Serve immediately or prepare up to one day in advance.

Chapter 16: Speedy Suppers

Fried Cauliflower Rice

Preparation time: 55 minutes

Cooking time: 10 minutes

Servings: 2

Ingredients:

- 1 piece Cauliflower

- 2 tablespoon Coconut oil

- 1 piece Red onion

- 4 cloves Garlic

- 60 ml vegetable broth

- 1 ½ cm fresh ginger

- 1 teaspoon Chili flakes

- ½ pieces Carrot

- ½ pieces Red bell pepper

- ½ pieces Lemon (the juice)

- 2 tablespoon pumpkin seeds

- 2 tablespoon fresh coriander

Directions:

1. Cut the cauliflower into small rice grains in a food processor.

2. Finely chop the onion, garlic, and ginger, cut the carrot into thin strips, dice the bell pepper and finely chop the herbs.

3. Melt 1 tablespoon of coconut oil in a pan and add half of the onion and garlic to the pan and fry briefly until translucent.

4. Add cauliflower rice and season with salt.

5. Pour in the broth and stir everything until it evaporates and the cauliflower rice is tender.

6. Take the rice out of the pan and set it aside.

7. Melt the rest of the coconut oil in the pan and add the remaining onions, garlic, ginger, carrots, and peppers.

8. Fry for a few minutes until the vegetables are tender. Season them with a little salt.

9. Add the cauliflower rice again, heat the whole dish, and add the lemon juice.

10. Garnish with pumpkin seeds and coriander before serving.

Minty Tomatoes and Corn

Preparation time: 10 minutes

Cooking time: 65 minutes

Servings: 2

Ingredients:

- 2 c. corn

- 1 tbsp. rosemary vinegar

- 2 tbsps. chopped mint

- 1 lb. sliced tomatoes

- ¼ tsp. black pepper

- 2 tbsps. olive oil

Directions:

1. In a salad bowl, combine the tomatoes with the corn and the other ingredients, toss and serve.

2. Enjoy!

Pesto Green Beans

Preparation time: 10 minutes

Cooking time: 55 minutes

Servings: 2

Ingredients:

- 2 tbsps. olive oil

- 2 tsps. sweet paprika

- Juice of 1 lemon

- 2 tbsps. basil pesto

- 1 lb. trimmed and halved green beans

- ¼ tsp. black pepper

- 1 sliced red onion

Directions:

1. Heat up a pan with the oil over medium-high heat, add the onion, stir and sauté for 5 minutes.

2. Add the beans and the rest of the ingredients, toss, cook over medium heat for 10 minutes, divide between plates and serve.

Scallops and Sweet Potatoes

Preparation time: 5 minutes

Cooking time: 22 minutes

Servings: 4

Ingredients:

- 1 pound scallops

- ½ teaspoon rosemary, dried

- ½ teaspoon oregano, dried

- 2 tablespoons avocado oil

- 1 yellow onion, chopped

- 2 sweet potatoes, peeled and cubed

- ½ cup chicken stock

- 1 tablespoon cilantro, chopped

Directions:

1. Heat up a pan with the oil over medium heat, add the onion and sauté for 2 minutes.

2. Add the sweet potatoes and the stock, toss and cook for 10 minutes more.

3. Add the scallops and the remaining ingredients, toss, cook for another 10 minutes, divide everything into bowls and serve.

Citrus Salmon

Preparation time: 10 minutes

Cooking time: 45 minutes

Servings: 2

Ingredients:

- 1 ½ lb. salmon fillet with skin on

- Salt and pepper to taste

- 1 medium red onion, chopped

- 2 tablespoons parsley, chopped

- 2 teaspoons lemon rind, grated

- 2 teaspoons orange rind, grated

- 2 tablespoons extra virgin olive oil

- 1 lemon, sliced thinly

- 1 orange, sliced thinly

- 1 cup vegetable broth

Directions:

1. Line your crockpot with parchment paper and top with the lemon slices.

2. Season salmon with salt and pepper and place it on top of the lemon.

3. Cover the fish with the onion, parsley, and grated citrus rinds, and oil over the fish. Top with orange slices, reserving a few for garnish.

4. Pour broth around, but not directly overtop your salmon.

5. Cover and cook on low for 2 hours.

6. Preheat oven to 400 degrees F.

7. When salmon is opaque and flaky, remove from the crockpot carefully using the parchment paper and transfer to a baking sheet. Place in the oven for 5 – 8 minutes to allow the salmon to brown on top.

8. Serve garnished with orange and lemon slices.

Mediterranean Paleo Pizza

Preparation time: 55 minutes

Cooking time: 25 minutes

Servings: 2

Ingredients:

For the pizza crusts:

- 120 g Tapioca flour

- 1 teaspoon Celtic sea salt

- 2 tablespoon Italian spice mix

- 45 g Coconut flour

- 120 ml Olive oil (mild)

- 120 ml Water (warm)

- 1 egg (beaten)

For covering:

- 2 tablespoon Tomato paste (can)

- ½ pieces Zucchini

- ½ pieces Eggplant

- 2 pieces Tomato

- 2 tablespoon Olive oil (mild)

- 1 tablespoon Balsamic vinegar

Directions:

1. Preheat the oven to 190 ° C and line a baking sheet with parchment paper.

2. Cut the vegetables into thin slices.

3. Mix the tapioca flour with salt, Italian herbs, and coconut flour in a large bowl.

4. Pour in olive oil and warm water and stir well.

5. Then add the egg and stir until you get an even dough.

6. If the dough is too thin, add 1 tablespoon of coconut flour at a time until it is the desired thickness. Always wait a few minutes before adding more coconut flour, as it will take some time to absorb the moisture. The intent is to get a soft, sticky dough.

7. Divide the dough into two parts and spread them in flat circles on the baking sheet (or make 1 large sheet of pizza as shown in the picture).

8. Bake in the oven for about 10 minutes.

9. Brush the pizza with tomato paste and spread the aubergines, zucchini, and tomato overlapping on the pizza.

10. Drizzle the pizza with olive oil and bake in the oven for another 10-15 minutes.

11. Drizzle balsamic vinegar over the pizza before serving.

Chapter 17: Easy Sirtfood Snacks

Kale Chips

Preparation time: 5 Minutes

Cooking time: 55 Minutes

Servings: 2

Ingredients:

- 1 large head of curly kale, wash, dry and pulled from stem

- 1 tbsp. extra virgin olive oil

- Minced parsley

- A squeeze of lemon juice

- Cayenne pepper (just a pinch)

- Dash of soy sauce

Directions:

1. In a large bowl, rip the kale from the stem into palm-sized pieces. Sprinkle the minced parsley, olive oil, soy sauce, a squeeze of lemon juice, and a very small pinch of cayenne powder. Toss with a set of tongs or salad forks, and make sure to coat all of the leaves.

2. If you have a dehydrator, turn it on to 118 F, spread out the kale on a dehydrator sheet, and leave it there for about 2 hours.

3. If you are cooking them, place parchment paper on top of a cookie sheet. Lay the bed of kale and separate it a bit to make sure the kale is evenly toasted. Cook for 10-15 minutes maximum at 250F.

Moroccan Leeks Snack

Preparation time: 5 minutes

Cooking time: 0 minutes

Servings: 3

Ingredients:

- 1 bunch radish, sliced

- 3 cups leeks, chopped

- 1 ½ cups olives, pitted and sliced

- Pinch turmeric powder

- 2 tablespoons essential olive oil

- 1 cup cilantro, chopped

Directions:

1. Take a bowl and mix in radishes, leeks, olives, and cilantro.

2. Mix well.

3. Season with pepper, oil, turmeric and toss well.

4. Serve and enjoy!

Honey Nuts

Preparation time: 5 Minutes

Cooking time: 35 Minutes

Servings: 2

Ingredients:

- 150g (5oz) walnuts

- 150g (5oz) pecan nuts

- 50g (2oz) softened butter

- 1 tablespoon honey

- ½ bird's-eye chili, very finely chopped and deseeded

Directions:

1. Preheat the oven to 180C/360F. Combine the butter, honey, and chili in a bowl, then add the nuts and stir them well. Spread the nuts onto a lined baking sheet and roast them in the oven for 10 minutes, stirring once halfway through. Remove from the oven and allow them to cool before eating.

Snack Bites

Preparation time: 5 Minutes

Cooking time: 35 Minutes

Servings: 2

Ingredients:

- 120g walnuts

- 30g dark chocolate (85% cocoa)

- 250g dates

- 1 tablespoon pure cocoa powder

- 1 tablespoon turmeric

- 1 tablespoon of olive oil

- Contents of a vanilla pod or some vanilla flavoring

Directions:

1. Coarsely crumble the chocolate and mix it with the walnuts in a food processor into a fine powder.

2. Then add the other ingredients and stir until you have a uniform dough. If necessary, add 1 to 2 tablespoons of water.

3. Form 15 pieces from the mixture and refrigerate in an airtight tin for at least one hour.

4. The bites will remain in the refrigerator for a week.

Herb Roasted Chickpeas

Preparation time: 5 minutes

Cooking time: 30 minutes

Servings: 3

Ingredients:

- 1 can of chickpeas, drained
- 1 - 2 tablespoon extra-virgin olive oil
- ½ teaspoon dried lovage
- ½ teaspoon dried basil
- 1 teaspoon garlic powder
- ⅛ teaspoon cayenne powder
- ¼ teaspoon fine salt

Directions:

1. Preheat oven to 400 degrees F and cover a large baking sheet with parchment paper.

2. Spread chickpeas out evenly over a pan in a single layer and roast for 30 minutes.

3. Remove from oven and transfer to a heat-resistant bowl.

4. Add the olive oil and toss to coat each chickpea. Sprinkle with herbs and toss again to distribute.

5. Return to oven for an additional 15 minutes.

6. Let cool for at least 15 minutes before eating.

Easy Seed Crackers

Preparation time: 10 minutes

Cooking time: 60 minutes

Servings: 2

Ingredients:

- 1 cup boiling water
- ⅓ cup chia seeds
- ⅓ cup sesame seeds
- ⅓ cup pumpkin seeds
- ⅓ cup Flaxseeds
- ⅓ cup sunflower seeds
- 1 tablespoon Psyllium powder
- 1 cup almond flour
- 1 teaspoon salt
- ¼ cup coconut oil, melted

Directions:

1. Preheat your oven to 300 degrees F.
2. Line a cookie sheet with parchment paper and keep it on the side.

3. Add listed ingredients (except coconut oil and water) to a food processor and pulse until ground.

4. Transfer to a large mixing bowl and pour melted coconut oil and boiling water, mix.

5. Transfer mix to a prepared sheet and spread into a thin layer.

6. Cut dough into crackers and bake for 60 minutes.

7. Cool and serve.

8. Enjoy!

Chapter 18: Top Sirt Desserts

Chocolate Balls

Preparation time: 5 Minutes

Cooking time: 25 Minutes

Servings: 2

Ingredients:

- 50g (2oz) peanut butter (or almond butter)

- 25g (1oz) cocoa powder

- 25g (1oz) desiccated (shredded) coconut

- 1 tablespoon honey

- 1 tablespoon cocoa powder for coating

Directions:

1. Place the ingredients into a bowl and mix. Using a teaspoon, scoop out a little of the mixture and shape it into a ball.

2. Roll the ball in a little cocoa powder and set it aside. Repeat for the remaining mixture. It can be eaten straight away or stored in the fridge.

Warm Berries & Cream

Preparation time: 5 Minutes

Cooking time: 45 Minutes

Servings: 2

Ingredients:

- 250g (9oz) blueberries

- 250g (9oz) strawberries

- 100g (3½ oz) redcurrants

- 100g (3½ oz) blackberries

- 4 tablespoons fresh whipped cream

- 1 tablespoon honey

- Zest and juice of 1 orange

Directions:

1. Place all of the berries into a pan along with the honey and orange juice. Gently heat the berries for around 5 minutes until warmed through. Serve the berries into bowls and add a dollop of whipped cream on top. Alternatively, you could top them off with fromage frais or yogurt.

Chocolate Fondue

Preparation time: 5 Minutes

Cooking time: 35 Minutes

Servings: 2

Ingredients:

- 125g (4oz) dark chocolate (min 85% cocoa)

- 300g (11oz) strawberries

- 200g (7oz) cherries

- 2 apples, peeled, cored, and sliced

- 100mls (3½ fl oz) double cream (heavy cream)

Directions:

1. Place the chocolate and cream into a fondue pot or saucepan and warm it until smooth and creamy. Serve in the fondue pot or transfer it to a serving bowl. Scatter the fruit on a serving dish ready to be dipped into the chocolate.

Mocha Chocolate Mousse

Preparation time: 5 Minutes

Cooking time: 35 Minutes

Servings: 2

Ingredients:

- 250g dim chocolate (85% cocoa solids)

- 6 medium unfenced eggs, isolated

- 4 tbsp solid dark espresso

- 4 tbsp almond milk

- Chocolate espresso beans to enrich

Directions:

1. Soften the chocolate in a huge bowl set over a skillet of delicately stewing water, ensuring the base of the bowl doesn't contact the water. Expel the bowl from the heat and leave the dissolved chocolate to cool to room temperature.

2. When the softened chocolate is at room temperature, race in the egg yolks each in turn and afterward tenderly overlap in the espresso and almond milk.

3. Utilizing a hand-held electric blender, whisk the egg whites until firm pinnacles structure, at that point blend several tablespoons into the chocolate blend to release it. Delicately overlap in the rest an enormous metal spoon.

4. Move the mousse to singular glasses and smooth the surface. Spread with stick film and chill for in any event 2 hours, preferably medium-term. Enliven with chocolate espresso beans before serving.

Walnut & Date Loaf

Preparation time: 5 Minutes

Cooking time: 45 Minutes

Servings: 2

Ingredients:

- 250g (9oz) self-rising flour

- 125g (4oz) Medjool dates, chopped

- 50g (2oz) walnuts, chopped

- 250mls (8fl oz) milk

- 3 eggs

- 1 medium banana, mashed

- 1 teaspoon baking soda

Directions:

1. Sieve the baking soda and flour into a bowl. Add in the banana, eggs, milk, and dates and combine all the ingredients thoroughly. Transfer the mixture to a lined loaf tin and smooth it out. Scatter the walnuts on top. Bake the loaf in the oven at 180C/360F for 45 minutes. Transfer it to a wire rack to cool before serving.

Chocolate Brownies

Preparation time: 5 Minutes

Cooking time: 35 Minutes

Servings: 2

Ingredients:

- 200g (7oz) dark chocolate (min 85% cocoa)
- 200g (70z) Medjool dates, stone removed
- 100g (3½oz) walnuts, chopped
- 3 eggs
- 25mls (1fl oz) melted coconut oil
- 2 teaspoons vanilla essence
- ½ teaspoon baking soda

Directions:

1. Place the dates, chocolate, eggs, coconut oil, baking soda, and vanilla essence into a food processor and mix until smooth. Stir the walnuts into the mixture. Pour the mixture into a shallow baking tray. Transfer to the oven and bake at 180C/350F for 25-30 minutes. Allow it to cool. Cut into pieces and serve.

Pistachio Fudge

Preparation time: 5 Minutes

Cooking time: 55 Minutes

Servings: 2

Ingredients:

- 225g (8oz) Medjool dates

- 100g (3½ oz) pistachio nuts, shelled (or other nuts)

- 50g (2oz) desiccated (shredded) coconut

- 25g (1oz) oats

- 2 tablespoons water

Directions:

1. Place the dates, nuts, coconut, oats, and water into a food processor and process until the ingredients are well mixed. Remove the mixture and roll it to 2cm (1 inch) thick. Cut it into 10 pieces and serve.

Spiced Poached Apples

Preparation time: 5 Minutes

Cooking time: 55 Minutes

Servings: 2

Ingredients:

- 4 apples

- 2 tablespoons honey

- 4 star anise

- 2 cinnamon sticks

- 300mls (½ pint) green tea

Directions:

1. Place the honey and green tea into a saucepan and bring to a boil. Add the apples, star anise, and cinnamon. Reduce the heat and simmer gently for 15 minutes. Serve the apples with a dollop of crème fraîche or Greek yogurt.

Chapter 19: Smoothie Sirt

Kale and Blackcurrant Smoothie

Preparation time: 5 Minutes

Cooking time: 45 Minutes

Servings: 2

Ingredients:

- 2 teaspoons of honey

- 1 cup freshly made green tea

- 10 baby kale leaves

- 1 ripe banana

- 40g blackcurrants

- 6 ice cubes

Directions:

1. Prepare green tea and stir honey into it until dissolved.

2. Add all the ingredients into a blender and blend until smooth. Serve at once.

Strawberry & Beet Smoothie

Preparation time: 5 Minutes

Cooking time: 45 Minutes

Servings: 2

Ingredients:

- 2 cups frozen strawberries, pitted and chopped

- 2/3 cup frozen beets, chopped

- 1 teaspoon fresh ginger, peeled and chopped

- 1 teaspoon fresh turmeric, peeled and grated

- ½ cup fresh orange juice

- 1 cup unsweetened almond milk

Directions:

1. Add all ingredients into a high-power blender and pulse until smooth.

2. Pour the smoothie into two glasses and serve immediately.

Matcha Berries Smoothie

Preparation time: 5 Minutes

Cooking time: 45 Minutes

Servings: 2

Ingredients:

- 2 cups frozen mixed berries

- 2 Medjool dates, pitted

- ½ teaspoon fresh ginger, peeled and chopped

- 1 tablespoon chia seeds

- 2 cups unsweetened almond milk

Directions:

1. Add all ingredients into a high-power blender and pulse until smooth.

2. Pour the smoothie into two glasses and serve immediately.

Grapes & Rocket Smoothie

Preparation time: 5 Minutes

Cooking time: 50 Minutes

Servings: 2

Ingredients:

- 2 cups seedless green grapes

- 2 cups fresh rocket leaves

- 2 Medjool dates, pitted

- 1 teaspoon fresh lemon juice

- 1½ cups water

- 4 ice cubes

Directions:

1. Add all the ingredients into a high-power blender and pulse until creamy.

2. Pour the smoothie into two glasses and serve immediately.

Kale & Orange Smoothie

Preparation time: 5 Minutes

Cooking time: 45 Minutes

Servings: 2

Ingredients:

- 3 cups fresh kale leaves

- 1 large orange, peeled

- 2 teaspoons raw honey

- 2 cups unsweetened almond milk

Directions:

1. Add all ingredients into a high-power blender and pulse until smooth.

2. Pour the smoothie into two glasses and serve immediately.

Chapter 20: The Sirtfood Green Juice

Celery Juice

Preparation time: 25 Minutes

Cooking time: 0 Minutes

Servings: 2

Ingredients:

- 8 celery stalks with leaves

- 2 tablespoons fresh ginger, peeled

- 1 lemon, peeled

- ½ cup filtered water

- Pinch of salt

Directions:

1. Add all ingredients in a blender and pulse until well combined.

2. Through a fine mesh strainer, strain the juice and transfer it into two glasses.

3. Serve immediately.

Orange & Kale Juice

Preparation time: 15 Minutes

Cooking time: 0 Minutes

Servings: 2

Ingredients:

- 5 large oranges, peeled and sectioned

- 2 bunches of fresh kale

Directions:

1. Add all ingredients into a juicer and extract the juice according to the manufacturer's method.

2. Pour into two glasses and serve immediately.

Grape and Melon Juice

Preparation time: 15 Minutes

Cooking time: 0 Minutes

Servings: 2

Ingredients:

- ½ cucumber, peeled if preferred, halved, seeds removed and roughly chopped

- 1 oz young spinach leaves stalk removed

- 4 oz red seedless grapes

- 4 oz cantaloupe melon, peeled, deseeded, and cut into chunks

Directions:

1. Blend together in a juicer or blender until smooth.

Sirtfood Green Juice

Preparation time: 15 Minutes

Cooking time: 0 Minutes

Servings: 2

Ingredients:

- 10 g of flat-leaf parsley

- 4 large handfuls of kale (150g)

- 2 large handful of rockets (60g)

- 10 g of lovage leaves (optional)

- 300 g of green celery, the leaves

- 1 medium green apple

- 1 lemon

- 1 level teaspoon of matcha green tea

Directions:

1. Mix the parsley, kale, rocket, and lovage together and juice. Also, re-juice the remnants to end up with about 100ml of juice from the greens.

2. Juice the celery and apple. Then squeeze the lemon into the juice. The whole juice should give up to 500ml of juice in total. It may be slightly more.

3. Add the matcha green tea, stir vigorously, and serve. You can top up with water.

Conclusion

I hope this guide has helped you become acquainted with the Sirtfood diet and achieve your weight loss and health goals. Sirtuins strengthen the immune system, help build muscle, and ensure that cell metabolism decreases - in other words, the aging process is slowed down, you stay "young longer." All you need to do is switch to foods that activate many sirtuins.

The next step is to test out all of the recipes and follow along with each of the phases with the proper foods and drinks. Follow the two planned stages, Phase 1 and Phase 2, and you will be guaranteed to enjoy more energy, vitality, a lighter feeling, and on average, about 7 lbs. lighter on the scale each week.

Over the course of this book, you have seen the best sirtfood recipes you can try at home. By learning how to your meals, you will be able to easily master the sirtfood diet with little day-to-day effort required. You will be able to enjoy delicious meals at a moment's notice without having to struggle after a long day of work.

You can trust that the Sirt diet works, as many people have experienced a profound change from the plan. While you may have heard about Adele's fifty-pound loss, there are many less famous people around the world who have had similar success. Give phases one and two a try, just once, and you are sure to see results. If you can commit to trying it out for just those few weeks, then you can feel confident in either maintaining the plan through including sirtfoods in your regular diet. You might even repeat phases one and two for increased weight loss.

SIMPLY INTERMITTENT FASTING

FOR WOMEN

THE ULTIMATE STEP BY STEP GUIDE TO LIVING A HEALTHY
LIFESTYLE, BURN FAT AND HEAL YOUR BODY THROUGH THE SELF-
CLEANSING PROCESS OF AUTOPHAGY

Josie Kidd

INTRODUCTION

If you are an early bird, being most productive early in the day and usually in bed when the sun goes down, you can choose to eat earlier, say from 9 am – 5 pm. For all the night owls out there who see midnight on a regular basis, pushing your eating window back to 4 pm – 12 am is no problem at all. Any way you design your intermittent fasting plan is fine, so long as you follow the foundational rules: no calories during your fasting period (while still staying properly hydrated) and sticking to consuming all of your calories during the strict eating window that you designate.

If this is the first time you hear about intermittent fasting, you may be ready to close it immediately and never even consider this lifestyle. If that is you, this feeling is probably due to outdated fitness and nutrition advice that society and so-called "gurus" have hammered into your mind for decades. You have without a doubt heard that breakfast is the most important meal of the day, or eating 5-6 small meals every 2-3 hours throughout the day is the most effective way for efficient metabolism, or that 'starving' yourself in an attempt to lose weight is counterproductive, etc.

Before we even begin to debunk these myths with all of the benefits of intermittent fasting, you need to realize that this is not a new concept by any means. Eating throughout the course of the entire day is a relatively new concept. Food has become so convenient and accessible in today's society that we are trained into believing we need three square meals a day. Society is so concerned with eating, instant gratification of our dietary desires that there are fast-food restaurants on every corner with their flashing neon signs advertising the latest $5 calorie bomb. Is it any surprise then that obesity levels are soaring, heart disease and stroke are running rampant, and people are unhealthier than ever before?

From our earliest ancestors all the way up until a few hundred years ago, the habit of eating one large meal at the end of the day was the norm. Ancient humans were hunter-gatherers, spending the entire day foraging for edible vegetation, hunting game, and just trying to survive. Eating was considered a celebratory ritual and was accompanied by a feast each evening when the food was brought back to the tribe. Even our modern ancestors spent their days farming the land, working whatever job needed to be done for their families, eating one large meal after a hard day's work.

While I am by no means saying that these people had it better than we do now (I would rather eat a few too many calories each day than have to survive a saber-toothed tiger attack), they did in fact reap many of the benefits of intermittent fasting without even realizing it. To digress, eating throughout the duration of the day is a relatively new concept that is not at all necessary to a healthy lifestyle.

CHAPTER 1: WHAT IS INTERMITTENT FASTING?

Relying on the knowledge of ancient cultures grants a certain amount of philosophical insight but is limited in the scientific background our twenty-first-century minds require to be safe. Fortunately, many studies on IF are popping up all over the Internet, with sound scientific evidence that fasting is as safe and effective, if not more so than any other diet that hits the mainstream. For decades, we have thought that what we eat is the most important aspect of whether or not our diets are considered healthy. However, many other factors are in play. Not only what we eat, but how it's prepared, where it's sourced, and when we eat. These combined with physical and mental exercise create our state of health, and IF affects all of these aspects.

BENEFITS AND SIDE EFFECTS OF INTERMITTENT FASTING

By taking on an IF routine, we funnel our view of food and meals through a new lens, thus transforming our mindset about food and the food we ingest and when. This transformation has been shown to increase self-worth while simultaneously reduce stress, which on a psychological level is incredibly beneficial for someone looking to lose weight. Let's keep this positive outlook and confidence in mind as we approach IF from a strictly scientific perspective.

In a very broad sense, IF's physical results are attributed to calorie restriction. It makes sense, right? Eat less, get thin. But it goes deeper than this simple equation. Lab studies have shown that calorie restriction has been attributed to the reduction of illnesses related to death and lengthened lifespans. Studies have shown that in mice obesity, the risk of metabolic diseases is lowered due to caloric restriction – these reactions have been proven to translate to humans. Not only can the restrictions help prevent obesity, but they were also shown to reset circadian rhythms and balance the rhythm of hormonal secretions. These rhythms, of which there are many, keep our body in check, ensuring that our body is running smoothly and efficiently. This biological rhythm is very apparent when a fast begins. The rhythm of your digestive system becomes very clear while fasting. Since digestion is essentially 'turned off' once we go to bed, it is subsequently turned back on the moment we intake calories the next morning. So, if we restrict calorie intake, our digestive system will rest until we eat again; while it rests, it repairs itself. By giving our systems plenty of time to repair in between meals, we achieve a simple yet effective and concise practice that assists our body with its natural healing methods. With IF and assigning a strict consumption window, we can actively engage with our natural digestive rhythm, keeping it in sync with the rest of our body as we see fit. The digestive system seems to be an obvious player in weight loss, but what about the control center and epic organ, the human brain?

The human brain is mysterious and complicated; science has certainly only scratched the surface of what must be an infinite amount of investigation into the brain. As the 'control center' of our entire body, it plays a major role in weight loss. The brain not only influences the physical aspects of the body, hormone regulation, and autonomous actions like breathing and blood pumping, but also more in-depth metaphysical ideas, like thought and emotion, are considered to be housed in the brain to some extent. As mysterious as it is, we will stand with these claims. And so, our ideas will play a huge role in our IF journey, and a positive outlook and practicing confidence-building affirmations will go hand in hand with the fasting experience. So consider the brain an avenue for thought and emotion. You are in control, and IF will help you come to this realization.

We've spent our whole lives thinking and believing that the societal structure of diets and foods are the most efficient. We need to break from these patterns and do what is best for us individually. Again, no one way of living will work for everyone. On the scientific level, we send signals to our brain that allow it to regulate and restore where need be. So, naturally, if you were to eat less or not eat when you normally do, the brain will assume that the food is scarce and will take the necessary actions. Although the brain may reduce the metabolic rate and attempt to conserve fat reserves, it is still burning reserved fat instead of recently ingested sugars, combined with suitable exercise (found later in the book). This is a very effective and safe weight loss strategy. However, let's not forget that the brain will also start releasing growth hormones to regulate and account for new changes in diet and routine. These are hormones that have been shown to increase longevity and reduce the effects of aging. The brain isn't the only organ that responds positively to IF.

Many wonder about the idea of the heart being the center of love and emotion. The symbolic idea of the heart is timeless, but what role can it play in our IF journey? The heart regulates blood flow, then the blood distributes nutrients and antibodies to all parts of the body. Considering the major causes of heart disease – cholesterol, blood pressure, weight, and diabetes – we find studies that show how IF assists in balancing all these bodily functions. The influence that this kind of fasting can have on these functions is important. As mentioned before, IF can help reset and assist the body to heal naturally. So, in turn, fasting helps regulate and balance these functions, then fasting directly influences the heart and its major enemies. We will discuss later in the book the potential risks of fasting, but here, we would like to state that some cases have found that extensive fasting can be attributed to electrolyte imbalances, which could affect the heart in negative ways.

The third major organ we want to focus on is the liver. The liver acts as a filtration system for the body while also producing bile to be sent to the intestines. As the filtration system, the liver will play a key role in the positive effects of IF. The caloric restriction itself acts as a symbolic representation of purification while quite literally not consuming any foods for a prolonged period will assist the liver in repairing itself. One particular study also shows us that when calories are restricted, the liver secretes a protein that adjusts the liver's metabolism. The regulation of the metabolism is key in producing weight loss results, and as we've seen, fasting interacts with the metabolism on many levels.

The science that has dedicated itself to fasting has shown what many believed for centuries before computers – that fasting is an all-around beneficial practice for overall wellbeing. Along with the three major organs discussed above, some key points should be emphasized:

- It gives the body more energy by assisting in the creation of mitochondria, which are power sources within every cell of your body. This gives you the energy that is used throughout the body. Having more energy will only assist in keeping up regular exercise and daily duties.

- It boosts growth hormone secretions in the brain. Although available in supplements, wouldn't human growth hormones (HGH) be more effective naturally occurring in the brain? By fasting, we increase the levels secreted by the brain, thus taking advantage of the hormone's natural ability to slow the effects of aging, improve cognitive performance, and protect the brain's health overall.

- It and its caloric restrictions allow the body to burn up stored fat rather than sugars. Fat is a cleaner source of energy than carbs or sugars and reduces inflammation by lowering free radical production, and free radicals are thought to oxidize cells, which could lead to autoimmune diseases and the like.

- It reduces inflammation, which is attributed to many common diseases, such as dementia and obesity. Inflammation damages cells and IF helps to clean away the damaged cells. Ketones are produced through the burning of fat instead of sugar, and they regulate inflammation. IF also helps the body not become resistant to insulin. Insulin can potentially build up in the blood and create inflammation.

With the incredible effects that IF presents, it is no wonder that it was common amongst our ancestors and now common in the mainstream during the twenty-first century. We know through this science that IF can help us on so many levels, but what about our main goal with this book – weight loss? If we are to focus on shedding some pounds, we need to look deeper into the specific effects that this kind of fasting has on our excess fat and body image as a whole.

The Intermittent Fasting system has many undeniable advantages. Some of them are even confirmed by scientific studies.

However, Intermittent Fasting, especially if you have health problems, should be practiced only after consulting with your doctor. Otherwise, there is a risk of developing problems with the gastrointestinal tract and other organs.

POSITIVE ASPECTS

Intermittent Fasting teaches self-control. Over time, a person learns to distinguish true hunger from the psychological need to chew something.

Slow rates of fat burning are compensated by a guarantee of stable results.

The advantage of Intermittent Fasting is also in the fact that recovery processes are activated. The body replaces damaged cells with new, healthy ones.

Scientists from Southern California in 2014 published an article claiming that the cells of the defense system regenerate better during periods of hunger strike. The body tries to save energy and recycles damaged cells of the immune system. During fasting, the number of old leukocytes decreases, but after eating food, new ones are produced, and the number returns to normal.

Five main benefits of this diet:

1. During the diet, you do not need to give up your favorite foods.

There are only recommendations that you should not overeat, lean on sweets and fast carbohydrates. Naturally, losing weight on donuts and chocolate bars has not been possible for anyone. But the only strict ban – sweets and soda. Eating very expensive delicacies and delights are not about this diet. Concentrate on foods that are enriched: protein (fish, meat, and cheese), fiber (spinach, broccoli, and asparagus), healthy fats (avocados, nuts).

2. Do not have to starve, because you need to eat food as much as five times a day.

Anyone with a diet is aware, the more times you eat, the smaller the portion. Indeed, by eating more times we set up our metabolic processes and do not torment ourselves with hunger. For a snack, eat yogurt with fruit and a salad with nuts.

3. You do not need to exhaust yourself with trainers.

Intermittent Fasting again has an advantage. It is recommended to spend 7 minutes a day on morning exercises. In addition, no hour of functional training in the gym! However, if you have a subscription, do not throw exercises, because the effect will only increase.

4. You decide on your meal schedule.

The main thing is that all meals fall within a period of eight hours. If the first time you ate at 10 am, then dinner after six is not recommended. Do not forget that the meal schedule should not differ much from day to day. The key to any effective diet is mode.

5. On the eight-hour diet, you can drink coffee and some wine!

The bans on coffee and alcohol are found in almost every diet, but not in the eight-hour diet, which makes it even nicer. Do not forget that in addition to your favorite lattes or Arabica and cocktails, you need to drink lots and lots of water

NEGATIVE ASPECTS OF INTERMITTENT FASTING

Adhering to such a diet, it is difficult to quickly gain muscle mass.

Fasting can affect the psychological state in different ways. Often it causes irritability, loss of concentration, and dizziness.

Fasting is contraindicated in several diseases: pancreatitis, tumors, respiratory diseases, and circulatory system diseases, diabetes mellitus, bodyweight deficiency, cardiac abnormalities, liver problems, thrombophlebitis, and thyrotoxicosis.

Some physiologists believe that starvation helps burn not fat but amino acids. A deficiency of protein leads to the destruction of collagen in muscle fibers. The absence of glucose in the body during the day triggers irreversible dystrophic processes.

Increases the likelihood of gallstones and kidney stones. Diabetics, as a result of fasting which lasts more than 12 hours, increases the risk of falling into a hypoglycemic coma.

As already mentioned, all individually. In addition, most of the disadvantages are associated with prolonged periods of hunger strike, and not with the regime at 12 o'clock, of which 7–9 fall asleep.

CHAPTER 2: INTERMITTENT FASTING AND AUTOPHAGY

Intermittent fasting is one of the best ways to detoxify your body, and it all happens through a process called autophagy. This process involves your body eating itself, cleaning damaged cells out of the way, removing toxins, and regenerating shiny new cells that are a great deal healthier.

As time passes, our cells gather in an awful lot of rubbish – damaged proteins, dead organelles, and oxidized particles that do nothing more than clogging up the way our bodies work. This leads to faster aging, hastens the onset of dementia, and increases the risk of some cancer, along with many other conditions related to age. Although some of our cells will replace themselves, many don't, and these need to last for as long as we last so, to help out, the body came up with its own way of getting rid of the crap and building up a defense system against disease.

HOW AUTOPHAGY WORKS

Try to imagine your body as your kitchen. Once you have prepared and cooked a meal, you clean up; the leftovers get tossed, and some food will be recycled. When you get up the next morning, your kitchen is clean. This is what autophagy does in your body.

Now consider the exact same scenario but 20 years later. Everything is older and not working quite so efficiently. When you finished your meal, you don't clean up quite so well as you used to. Some stuff gets thrown in the garbage, but some linger, hanging around clogging up everything.

The garbage doesn't get put out; instead, toxic waste begins building up in the kitchen; food ferments on the floor, and there are all kinds of indescribably nasty smells. And because of all the toxins and the pollutants, you struggle to keep up. This is autophagy not working as it should do in your body.

Normally, autophagy will buzz along quite nicely in the background, carrying out maintenance duties. When your body comes under high stress, autophagy kicks up a notch or two, protecting the body, and one of the periods of stress is famine. When autophagy is activated, the aging process is slowed, inflammation is reduced, and your body can cope with normal functioning. To help fight against disease and live longer, you need to push your autophagic response into a higher gear more naturally, and I'll tell you more about that in a while.

THE SCIENCE OF AUTOPHAGY

Over time, the human race has evolved, and now we live longer because our response to biological stressors is better. Much of this comes from the minuscule adaptations in p62, a protein that induces autophagy.

P62 can sense metabolic byproducts that cause damage to cells (known as ROS – reactive oxygen species) and activate itself so that the autophagic process begins. More specifically, these proteins remove the rubbish that accumulates in your body, giving you a better chance of handling those biological stresses, and it is this that keeps you healthy and young.

The result of autophagy that works well is homeostasis, or balanced functioning of the cells, along with great health. The rubbish is moved, and new cells form, and this leads to other benefits of the process, including slower aging, prevention or delay of neurodegenerative diseases, a reduction in inflammation, and a much better ability to function at peak performance. Oh, and did I mention it gives you a great skin complexion too? Detoxification at its best.

The big question is, once you kick the autophagic process into high gear, how soon will you see the results? Well, you should begin to benefit from it within a couple of weeks, but that will depend entirely on how you get it working properly.

3 WAYS TO KICKSTART AUTOPHAGY

There are a few ways to turn the process up, and none of them have anything to do with fast detox juices or cleanses. If you want to detox your body, clean your cells, reduce inflammation and so on, follow these tips;

EAT LCHF

A low carb, high-fat diet is important in the autophagic process because fat has to be the dominant macronutrient. It is much different from protein, which can transform into carbohydrates and then into sugar – fat can't do that. The ketogenic diet is one of the best when it comes to autophagy, and it works by burning fat instead of glucose as energy, mimicking a fasted state, and this kick starts the process naturally. Oh, and by the way, a low-carb high-fat diet works wonderfully with intermittent fasting.

PROTEIN FASTS

One or two days out of the week cut back your protein consumption to between 15 and 25 grams per day. This provides your body with a day in which to recycle those proteins, and this reduces inflammation and detoxes the cells without the loss of any muscle. Autophagy is triggered, and your body will turn to its own toxins and proteins and consume them – a great result.

TRY INTERMITTENT FASTING

By confining your meals to a set window of time each day, the autophagic process is naturally increased. Like the protein fast, intermittent fasting provides your body with a chance to catch the toxins and clean them out.

All of these three can be done together but, you do need to bear in mind that if you don't do intermittent fasting properly, it can cause an imbalance of hormones in women. To get around this, you should consume a breakfast that consists of fat only, like avocado or coffee made with butter and oil (Bulletproof coffee). By doing this, your body stays in a fasting state, and the fat tells the body and the brain that you are full.

CHAPTER 3: HEALTHIER WAY TO LOSE WEIGHT

There are so many different reasons why we all gain weight. Some people think everyone that is obese sits around eating junk all day. Sure, maybe some do this, but in general, there is usually an underlying health reason that someone might have struggled in trying to lose weight and reduce their overall weight gain.

As we mentioned earlier, when you are overweight, it will be even harder for you to try and reduce that weight and easier for your body to start to pack on even more pounds. One of the reasons that you might have trouble losing weight is because of your body's natural tendency to retain water.

CAUSE OF WEIGHT GAIN

If you are eating foods that are high in salt, then this can cause your body to hold on to a lot of weight through excess water. This will usually show itself in visual places, such as your chin/chest, your feet, or your hands. When you first start on a healthy diet, you might drop 20 pounds in as quickly as a month.

This is because your body is letting go of that water. Then, as weight loss progresses, it becomes a lot slower, because you're not holding onto that water. This can be very discouraging for some. They might start a drastic diet, losing five pounds in just a week. Then, however, they might gain back three pounds the next week and think that the diet doesn't work, quitting, and moving on. Always remember water retention in the struggle for weight loss.

Our bodies can sometimes resist our attempts at weight loss as well. If you are participating in extreme diets like only drinking lemon water for a week, but then go back to eating unhealthily next week, you're confusing your body. It will resist that diet in the first place in order to better deal with the fluctuations you're seeing. This is why you might feel like you gain weight quickly, or why if you lose weight, it doesn't always stay off.

Another cause of weight gain can be not eating right, along with exercising. You might be an active person or know an active person who frequently works out or participate in sports. Despite their dedication, they're still overweight. The biggest reason for this is unhealthy eating. Some people can get away with eating unhealthily and exercising and still having a low body weight and fit physique. However, for the most part, it's crucial that we also focus on healthier diets in addition to whichever workout we choose to add.

Alternatively, some people think they don't have to exercise at all, and the weight will just come off. In the beginning, this is true. If you don't work out and don't eat healthily, but then start to eat healthy food, you will lose some weight. You will eventually plateau, however, especially after your stomach and metabolism adjust. Not everyone has to dedicate an hour a day to the gym. However, light and frequent cardio, such as a walk every other day or 20 minutes on the treadmill a day, is still very important if you want to lose weight continually.

There are many sneaky foods that will get into our diets and cause us to hang onto unwanted weight as well. The biggest hidden food is sugar. This will often be found in highly processed foods. Some things might market themselves as organic, making you think "healthy." They might also show pictures of fruits and veggies, stating things like "contains two whole apples, one berry, one banana, etc." What they won't put on the front, however, is that they also contain %30 of your daily recommended sugar!

Things like yogurt, deli meats, frozen veggies, and other processed foods that are seemingly harmless might very well contain high levels of sodium, which will cause water retention, and high levels of sugar, which can imbalance your hormones and cause a higher amount of fat to be stored throughout your body.

Dehydration is another culprit of obesity. Water needs to be consumed in certain amounts depending on your body weight, regardless if you drink other beverages. Some people might think that they had some coffee, juice, tea, or even a soda and think this counts towards their hydration level. However, some of these will contain things that can even dehydrate you further, so it's crucial that you never deprive yourself of an excessive amount of water.

One of the biggest reasons that we might struggle with obesity and the overall ability to lose weight is because of the mentality around dieting. To lose weight doesn't mean to give up food for a month, and then the pounds come off and stay off. There's no pill, shake, or surgery that will help you stay in shape. These things will remove fat, but they won't keep them off and can end up causing you to gain more weight later on because of the intense fluctuation in debt we're giving our bodies. If you really want to lose weight and fight obesity, then we need to work with our body's natural fat-burning properties.

A HEALTHY AND BALANCED DIET

Fasting is a great way to lose weight. However, if you are eating unhealthy during the periods that you do eat, then fasting isn't going to end up doing you any good. Your body will eventually balance out.

You should be eating a balanced diet even if you read this book through and then decide fasting isn't for you. The combination of both, along with exercise, is going to be your secret to melting your body fat, however. Throughout this chapter, we are going to take a look at some of the best ways that you can burn your body fat through a healthy and balanced diet.

The biggest mistake dieters will make is by purchasing and focusing only on "diet," "organic," "natural," and other types of foods that are only labeled for being healthy. Don't be misguided by some fancy wording, especially blank statements like "part of a complete meal." Any meal could be complete! "Part of a healthy meal" is something that is actually saying something of value.

Start by cutting out as many processed foods as possible. We'll all have those pizza cravings after a night out at the bar or want to indulge in a sugary coffee with our breakfasts. However, you should be putting an emphasis on having these things as treats. If you have them every once in a while, your body will be able to process them easier, meaning it's not like you'll gain two pounds from having one slice of cake. However, if you have a slice of cake every day, you will start to gain weight again. Don't think you have to cut them out of your life altogether – this is the kind of all or nothing thinking that can send us into a panic and want to binge.

Of course, you might struggle with your control over food and find it difficult to have "just a few" of certain kinds of sweets. Still, make it a priority to reduce the number of junk food items you add in regularly.

Choose whole-wheat over white carbs, such as whole-wheat bread versus white bread, whole-grain pasta over white pasta, and so on. Pick lean meat like chicken and fish over heavier red meat like bacon and steak.

Pick fresh fruits and veggies over canned, and make sure if you do buy frozen that there are no additives. Always check your labels and make sure the sugar, salt, and fat content are lower than other vitamin and mineral counts that might be labeled.

Don't think you can't snack either. Smaller meals combined with healthier snacks throughout the day are always a better choice than just three huge meals.

REGULATING YOUR METABOLISM

The reason that some people will include cheat days in their diet is first to alleviate some of the pressures of dieting and give into their biggest cravings. It's also helpful in keeping your metabolism on its toes. Combined with fasting, this will help keep your metabolism active and regulated rather than sticking to one diet and one kind of food all the time.

Your metabolism is based on weight, age, and sex. The younger you are, the bigger you are, and the more muscles you have, the faster you burn food. Men typically have more muscles than women (think hips/breasts/and other fatty areas on women), which is why it might be easier for a husband to lose weight after giving up soda, while his wife struggles to lose a pound even though she eats nothing but salad. The combination of a balanced diet with fasting will help to keep your metabolism regulated.

HOW TO USE FASTING FOR WEIGHT LOSS

All of this means that adding fasting to whatever else you are doing will help you to lose weight. The more of these healthy habits you can add to your life, such as focusing on balanced meals and exercise, the better results you will see.

Fasting can burn fat, detoxify your body, and help build self-control. All of this can lead to the healthier lifestyle you've been looking for.

CHAPTER 4: TECHNIQUES OF INTERMITTENT FASTING

Before getting started with anything, make sure that you are fully prepared. You don't ever want to jump into a fast, because this is when unhealthy measures might be taken. It's highly encouraging to have a journal or notebook that you keep with you, and that can track your progress.

You will also want to do a trial period. Never think that your first fast is going to be "the one." Please don't get it in your head that everything will go perfect the first time around. It very well might, but if you expect perfection, you will get disappointed when things don't go right. When this occurs within a diet plan, it can lead to discouragement and the desire to give up altogether.

Of course, before getting started, ensure that you have spoken to a medical professional as well if you are worried about any other aspect of your health or if you have a history of health conditions that could be affected by fasting. For example, even a kidney issue might be affected, but a broken knee in the second grade likely won't play a part in your fasting plan.

KINDS OF INTERMITTENT FASTS AND BEST PRACTICES FOR WOMEN

As much as we remind ourselves throughout our lives that we can do anything men can, we do have to remember that we have different biological makeups. Of course, every woman and every man are different from each other regardless of sex and gender.

However, it's important to remember that the biological makeup of females is different from the biological makeup of men, meaning that it might be harder for our bodies to go through some of the same things that men will go through.

Some science even suggests that intermittent fasting won't offer as many benefits to women as men, but again, these are situational. For example, there was an isolated study that proved blood sugar to be more unmanageable in the first three weeks of women studied, but not men.

While kinds of studies like these do remind us of some of the cautions we face because of our biology, we have to remember that what doesn't work for some works for others and vice versa.

Women can be more sensitive to caloric changes in their diet, with some women finding that this can even stop or prolong their menstrual cycle. The reason for this happening can sometimes be due to the hypothalamus of the brain being affected during fasting.

A hormone called GnRH, which helps regulate various reproductive hormones, is disrupted by the changes in the hypothalamus, meaning that hormonal changes are going to affect your menstrual cycle. This could cause annoying periods, but even more serious; it could affect infertility, if that's something that you are concerned about now or down the line (Martin, 2008).

All of this information might seem frightening and could even make intermittent fasting seem less attractive as something that you might consider. However, have no fear!

It's important to know these things so that you know what not to do and the risks involved before doing anything. If you have a history of hormonal imbalances, such as irregular and infrequent menstrual cycles, endometriosis, PCOS, and other female-related health conditions, then you absolutely should discuss intermittent fasting with a professional before getting started.

Intermittent fasting could help to regulate these hormones and could be the solution to a preexisting condition. You might have irregular cycles due to poor health, and intermittent fasting could be the solution to help control your diet. However, it could also be something that disrupts these hormonal imbalances further, so consider the potential effects before getting started.

In order to prevent intermittent fasting from affecting you too much, you might try adding a multivitamin specifically for reproductive health to your diet. You can also look for ways to include more estrogen, such as through tofu/other soybean products, in natural and healthy ways.

WHAT YOU NEED TO KNOW ABOUT HUNGER

Before getting started with intermittent fasting, it's important that you have a good idea of what hunger really is. Of course, you've felt it since you could remember. You first feel it in your tummy, knowing that it's time to think about eating. Your stomach might make a noise, then maybe you get a headache, or your mood turns sour.

All of these things are signs that our body is using to tell us to eat. The thing is, our body doesn't know the difference between right now and an hour from now. We grow to realize that we'll make it another hour if we wait to eat, but our stomachs won't always take this change as easily.

When a baby is hungry, it cries until it gets fed. How many times have you seen, or as a parent experienced, moments where you wanted to say, "Can't you just wait five more minutes?" Babies don't know, and our stomachs can still function in the same way.

The best way to distract yourself from the initial hunger pains and desire to eat is to find a specific distraction you can do with your hands and your body, not just your mind. For example, you might think that you can watch TV, but your mind will still wander, and you might be thinking about the food you want to eat.

Physically remove yourself from where you are once you realize you're hungry. If you're sitting on the couch during a fast and you want to eat, go somewhere else. Take a shower, go for a walk, take a nap, or do whatever else you have to in order to keep your hands and your mind occupied so that no part of you is thinking about eating.

Remember that the hunger will pass as well. You won't spend the entire fast feeling like you're starving. Eventually, your body will start to burn fat, and you'll get that little boost of energy so that you won't feel the need to eat.

SIDE EFFECTS AND CAUTIONS WHILE MAKING THE TRANSITION TO INTERMITTENT FASTING

Intermittent fasting isn't the easiest thing you'll ever do, especially in the beginning. It's easy in concept, but five minutes hungry can sometimes feel like the end of the world! Remember to power through, as this feeling will fade. There are other side effects that you should be knowledgeable of before getting started with this diet as well.

Especially in women, there might be moments of mood swings, trouble focusing, lethargy, and headaches when you first get started (Whiteman, 2015). Have plenty of water, celery, carrots, coffee, and tea when you get started. Of course, avoid using any honey or sweetener in these drinks, but if you have to, have a couple of carrots or celery sticks instead of giving in completely when you feel moments of cravings. It's preferred to not eat anything, especially because eating a small amount might end up making you hungrier.

However, eating a couple of carrots is going to be way better than giving up on the fast and binging on junk food.

Don't keep these tempting foods in your house either. It might be hard when you have other members in the house who will want to keep them around but do your best to encourage family members or roommates to support you in the shopping as well as giving up some extra junk lying around the house.

The biggest thing you should remember when fasting is to be considerate of any eating disorders you might have. Anorexia, bulimia, and binge eating disorders are among the most common that many women might have struggled with in the past.

Fasting might not work for you first and foremost if you have a history of binging and purging because your body has become accustomed to this kind of eating pattern. If it's been a while since you struggled with an eating disorder, you can try, but be cautious of it triggering you back into old patterns.

A binge eating disorder can make it harder to start fasting, as well. If you are cutting off all foods too quickly, it might trigger you to want to binge right away.

Of course, you shouldn't be discouraged from trying these methods if you have had an eating disorder before, you need to be cautious. If the disorder has been professionally treated and you've come up with methods to prevent yourself from falling back into these kinds of behaviors, then you are at less of a risk than if the disorder occurred recently.

Practice in small ways, maybe with a four or five hour fast a day to ensure that no triggers are going to be run into while trying this diet out in the long-term.

HOW TO START INTERMITTENT FASTING

To actually get started, make sure that you have everything you will need during the fast. Then, when it comes to the eating periods, keep your fridge stocked. Though you might not be eating for a day, you want the food there the next day prepped and ready so that you won't be tempted to get takeout or order delivery. You might be tired of your fasting, so a meal already made and ready to eat in the fridge can help ensure you stay on track.

Keep your house accessible for a ton of water consumption as well. Keep pre-filled water jugs in the fridge if you like cold water, so you always have something to drink. Have ice cubes, big clean cups, and maybe even lemon in order to ensure that drinking water will be encouraged.

LEARN WHAT YOUR NATURAL EATING PATTERN IS

Before your fast, and even while it is happening, keep track of every moment you are hungry and all the times that you eat. This is going to be to help you learn what your natural eating pattern is. The more aware you are of the times that you want to eat the most, the easier it will be to combat some feelings of hunger and cravings.

Don't just keep track of when you feel like eating. Differentiate between times that you actually feel the hunger physically through stomach growling or headaches. Then, keep track of the biggest craving moments, times where you don't have to eat at all, but the moments that you want to sit there and snack.

Then, keep track of the times that you are actually eating. Then, you can look at this and make discoveries about your natural eating patterns. It will be easier to make intermittent fasting schedules based on these moments of wanting to eat, then.

START WITH AN EASIER FAST TRANSITION

Remember what we said previously – don't expect the first time to go exactly as planned. Someone who wants to build a castle will start with one brick at a time. If you want to eat an elephant, you do so bite by bite. Those who wish to move mountains will begin with the smallest pebble. All of these are old ideas about taking one step at a time.

Pick out a six-hour period that you are awake to try and fast. Maybe you stop eating at 4 pm for the day. Or perhaps you choose to wait to have your first meal until a late lunch. Whatever it is, just one time in a week, fast for this short period. This is going to help give you an idea of all the issues you might run into when you start to fast for real.

You might discover you're incredibly hungry beyond control. Perhaps a headache comes along, or you find a craving that you can't resist. Please keep track of these so you can come up with a plan to tackle these issues when they come to you during the real fast.

LISTEN TO YOUR BODY AND KNOW WHEN TO QUIT

You need food to eat, and that's just a fact. You could go on a vegan diet forever and be healthy all your life, but you couldn't fast forever. Eventually, your body would shut down because it would run out of energy!

Too much fasting can put your metabolic state out of whack, could lead to ketoacidosis, or have other long-term side effects. Like any diet, you have to consistently make the smart choices needed with your health in your best interest.

Part of this will be learning to listen to your body. This might seem easy, as we've been with our bodies all of our lives. However, it can sometimes be hard to tell what it really needs.

Have you ever declined an invitation to a party and felt guilty over it? It's not like you feel guilty for not going, but you might feel the guilt about skipping it. Though you have that bad feeling, it's hard to know what the real issue is behind it. Do you feel guilty about missing the party, or do you feel guilty because you had an obligation? In order to find this out, you have to look deep into yourself and question if what you are feeling is the reaction of emotion or if it is the true state of how things should be.

When it comes to dieting, you have to look inwards during these times as well. Sometimes you might feel a little nauseated and a potential headache. This might make you feel like something is really wrong or like you're dying. Really, this is a common side effect and not something that's worth ruining the diet over.

Alternatively, you might have a bad headache but ignore it and power through during a workout, not thinking twice. However, it could be a sign that you're dehydrated, as realized when you pass out in the gym locker room later on.

One symptom can have two different causes, and it can cause even more variant effects and reactions among different individuals. The best way to know if what you're doing is right or wrong is to listen to your body. When something doesn't feel right, trust it.

Just ensure to consistently check in with the difference between your mind and your body in terms of the signals that they might be giving you.

Remember to know when to quit as well. If you feel super sick, if you're losing weight rapidly, or if you don't feel like yourself anymore, it's a good time to take a break.

EAT HEALTHY IN BETWEEN

While you're eating during these intermittent fasting "off" moments, make sure that you are making healthier choices. We will discuss healthier foods to choose from while you're dieting, but remember the importance of including balanced, whole-food meals.

That can sound boring, as you might have thought before getting started that intermittent fasting means you can eat whatever you want! That might be how some people are able to do it, but not everyone will find the results they want with this method. If you really want to see the pounds come off, then you have to pair it with healthy eating.

There's another reason besides just the weight loss that healthy eating will be important. Aside from the way you physically feel, eating healthy will make you feel mentally better as well. This will help to keep the diet going longer.

For example, think about how hard it can be to stop eating chips once you start. It's harder not to eat a chip after you've already had one than it would be not to eat a chip at all. It can take a bit for our minds to catch up with our stomachs.

If you are eating unhealthy in between fasts, it will be much harder to stop, and it will be even harder to get started once again. Think of it as cleaning, working out, or doing anything else that requires a bit of work. It is so much harder if you take one hour of work and stretch it out amongst four hours than if you go for it and do it all at once. Think about how much longer a drive would be if you turned your car off and then on again at each stop sign or traffic light!

Once you get started, you'll want to make things as easy as possible. Keep up with a healthy lifestyle in your off days, and it will be easier to stick with the fast. At the same time, you want to ensure that your microbiome is being replenished. Balance your stomach back out with foods like antioxidant-rich berries, spinach, yogurt, fish, and other healthy foods that will make you feel balanced.

AVOID EXCESSIVE LEVELS OF SUGAR

The biggest thing you should focus on avoiding during your periods of eating off the fast are foods high in sugar. We already discussed that this is because your body will store the excess sugar as fat.

What's more challenging about this, however, is that it is something that could even be addictive. If you drink a sugary coffee drink every morning, or have soda for lunch, or do anything else ritualistic with sugar throughout your day, you can experience some withdrawal-like symptoms once you stop.

You might experience headaches, mood swings, and moments where you want to attack the most annoying person. If you are someone that has a lot of sugar in your life, then you might want to consider doing a sugar detox before fasting. Cold turkey is a great way to quit, but it's also very hard for many people to give up these things they might not have initially realized they were even addicted to in the first place.

Giving up sugar can be hard, but remember that things will taste so much better after you do! What's something sugary that you drink every day? For me, it's a caramel iced coffee, no matter where I go. After giving this up just for a week, when I went back to have a coffee, it was the sweetest thing I ever tasted! Let these things, like sweet iced coffee, become a treat and a reward, not a daily requirement!

CHAPTER 5: WHAT SHOULD YOU EAT AND WHAT NOT EAT

Before you start your first fast, however, it's helpful to know what's good to eat and drink versus what hurts the cause. This chapter is dedicated to that knowledge of what's good to eat and drink when Intermittent Fasting versus what to avoid at all costs.

10 GREAT FOODS TO EAT

When you're doing IF, you'll need to eat foods that give you enough energy to last until your next breakfast, and that can be tricky if you don't know what to look out for! This section lists 10 of the best foods to incorporate into your diet when practicing IF.

Avocado is high in calories and healthy fats, so it's perfect to have as a snack or in a meal.

Cruciferous vegetables like cauliflower, Brussel sprouts, broccoli, and more are full of fiber and so much more!

Potatoes of all kinds are great to satisfy one's hunger and provide a nutritional punch.

Legumes and beans of all varieties contain good carbohydrates that can help lower weight without too much restriction of calories.

Berries contain vitamin C, flavonoids, and antioxidants that will add a lot of good to your fast.

Eggs of any animal are packed with protein to help you build muscle and retain energy during the fast.

Wild-caught fish have a great amount of protein as well as vitamin D for one's brain and healthy fats and omega-3s for one's body.

Anything high in protein **or** high in probiotic content will be good to have along for the ride.

Grains and nuts are full of fiber and healthy fats for snacks or meals during your fast's eating windows.

Spices such as *cayenne pepper, psyllium husk, or dried dandelion* are natural weight loss agents that can help anyone's process.

3 FOODS TO AVOID

On the flip side, some foods will absolutely set you back on your path to progress, and it will be equally important to know what to steer clear of. The following list includes three foods to avoid at all costs.

Processed foods will be the most important things to avoid, especially as you prepare for your fast.

Highly GMO foods are also things to avoid when you're working through your fast. They can offset the actual nutrition being provided by other foods in your diet.

Sugary foods may curb your appetite, but they won't do anything good for your body in the long run. Steer clear for your future ease.

Moving forward, as we get ever closer to our goal of completely changing our outlook on the diet, we find ourselves with a bit of an appetite. But what foods are okay to eat while fasting? Although you could safely keep your normal diet and simply fast around it, we can optimize our transformation by including foods that are ideal to pair with a diet that includes regular Intermittent Fasting. With access to nearly any food we desire, it is tough not to grab the pizza slice or burger when we feel hungry. However, we're developing our confidence and control here, not simply fulfilling our immediate desires. By taking control of our instant desires, we empower ourselves to think mindfully of our next meal, and a dedicated IF regime assists us in accomplishing this life-altering goal.

First things first, let's take a moment to think about our diets. Go back one week and write out all the meals you had, including snacks and contemplate it:

- Were these foods I desired?

- Were these foods of convenience?

- Were there any foods that could have been easily left out?

- Were these foods rich in nutrients?

These questions are pretty straightforward, but let's try and be more abstract:

- Where did the food come from?

- Was this food natural?

- What time of the day was I eating?

- Was it a set routine?

- Why did I choose these particular foods?

- Was this the same diet I've maintained for over a decade?

This contemplation should be thorough and invigorating. There will be realizations and even more questions, more intimate ones. Let the thought process flow over you. This is a beginning step to being mindful of your diet. These simple questions will help prepare you for how your diet will change once IF begins. You will consciously change your habits, but you will also subconsciously be building a relationship with your desires and changing them from the inside out. Keep your diet in mind leading up to the fast and consider some options below if they haven't been in your diet before.

Many fad diets come and go over the years, but in reality, they are just that – fads. Cutting out carbs or only eating protein isn't going to give us the well-rounded, transformative effect we're searching for here. We need to balance our diet, explore nutrient-rich ingredients, and find alternatives to the ingredients that are most detrimental to our goals.

Moving forward, let us investigate what type of diets are best suited for IF. Since it requires you only to eat during certain parts of the day or only on certain days, we not only need to gorge ourselves on what we have in our hands, but also be aware of how balanced our meals are. Since we aim to lose weight while simultaneously transforming the way we view meals and food, we need meals and snacks that are mostly unprocessed, high in fiber, and have lean protein. But what we eat isn't the only factor. If you think about a 'normal' day of eating, you will realize that our digestive system is working from morning until night to digest three or more meals a day. This is just asking for weight gain since our stomachs are never empty, and our body doesn't need to burn our fat reserves for energy. So, we soon realize that the time we eat is also important. The timing will be covered in subsequent chapters.

As we think about raw, nutrient-rich food, we also consider where our food comes from. Foods produced locally will be richer in nutrients and promote the local economy by supporting smaller farms. This is a practice in mindfulness as we seek to develop a better relationship with food and, through this mindful notion, contribute to a more ecologically and economically balanced world around us. Since we seek to better ourselves through transformation, our relationship with food needs to be reevaluated, and an excellent place to start is where your food is sourced. You will also learn more about the foods available to you, educating yourself on which foods are in the season, thus helping you decide what foods you will be preparing during fasting weeks. Taking a visit to your local farmer's market is more than likely the best option for sourcing local foods, not to mention the relationship you build with other people who share the same notion of community support.

FOODS RICH IN NUTRIENTS IDEAL FOR A FASTING LIFESTYLE

LEAFY GREENS

Deep, dark, leafy greens are a staple in the optimized fasting diet. These foods are rich in vitamins A, C, and K, as well as plenty of potassium and fiber. These greens can replace the standard lettuce in any recipe and are available all year round. Kale, among many other leafy greens, is even considered one of the most nutrient-rich foods known to humans. If you are not a fan of the flavor of leafy greens, blend them up in a smoothie with some fruits to mask the taste. Some examples of delicious leafy greens include kale, spinach, collard greens, chard, turnip greens, and cabbage.

GARLIC

Garlic is found in many recipes and can be eaten raw if you don't mind the pungent flavor and aroma. High in B vitamins, vitamin C, calcium, copper, and selenium, this nutrient-rich food could potentially lower and balance blood pressure while also containing antibacterial and antifungal properties. Garlic can be a welcome ingredient in most meals, minced or whole.

POTATOES

Potatoes are versatile and fun to cook with. They pack a massive amount of potassium, copper, and iron while also containing a good amount of vitamins B and C. Another ideal factor for IF is how filling a potato can be. Try boiling potatoes for the most beneficial preparation method.

TOMATOES

With a wide variety of different types to choose from, tomatoes are versatile and yield many different flavors. Packed full of vitamins and minerals, these beautifully bright foods can be eaten raw by themselves or added to salads.

BROCCOLI

Notorious for being hated by many people, broccoli is full of vitamins C and K, among other vitamins and minerals. Best steamed or eaten raw in salads.

CAULIFLOWER

Cauliflower is an incredibly nutrient-rich food that deserves way more attention. Vitamin C, K, B12, and filled with fiber, this vegetable has much-needed minerals and small amounts of protein. Find creative recipes online or eat raw in salads.

SUNFLOWER SEEDS

An excellent source of vitamin E, these tiny seeds are great to snack on. Antioxidants, copper, phosphorous, and magnesium abound in these little seeds. Add to any salad or eat raw.

ALMONDS

Nuts and seeds are wonderful for snacking during IF. Almonds, in particular, pack a bunch of vitamin E, copper, magnesium and fiber. One downside is the large number of calories, so be cautious while on a restricted caloric intake and snacking on almonds.

BLUEBERRIES

Among the many berries and their many benefits, blueberries stand out when it comes to being rich in nutrients. Although not as rich in vitamins as most vegetables, blueberries boast a wild amount of antioxidants, which can protect the brain and repair cells. Throw some blueberries in a salad or snack on them raw.

RASPBERRIES

Although a little tough to find in some places, if you can get your hands on some raspberries, you can fulfill your body's needs for vitamin C, fiber, and manganese. Eat raw, with yogurt, or in smoothies.

CHOCOLATE

You're probably thinking of name brands of candy bars right now, but in all seriousness, dark chocolate is packed with antioxidants, fiber, iron, magnesium, and copper. Grabbing chocolate with 80% or higher cocoa content is the healthiest. Mix it with smoothies, nuts, or eat raw.

BEANS

Beans, black beans, in particular, are filled with iron and protein. They are filling and great to replace red meats for protein content that is much leaner. Plenty of minerals and folic acid come along with the versatile bean. Cook in chili, burritos, or even salads.

RICE

Among other whole grains, rice is rich in fiber and small amounts of vitamins and minerals. Rice is one of the most consumed foods in the world and can be mixed and paired with almost anything. Sweet or savory, rice goes a long way when fasting. It is filling, inexpensive, and easy to cook. Pair with sautéed vegetables, fish, tofu, and beans.

TOFU

Fermented soybean doesn't sound appealing to everyone, but tofu is incredibly versatile and is a great source of lean, plant-based protein. As a great alternative to red meats and other animal proteins, tofu is a lynchpin in a vegetarian or vegan diet. Marinate and sauté with veggies or press and fry for sandwiches.

SALMON

Salmon stands out among fish as a nutrient-rich powerhouse. Filled with omega-3 fatty acids and plenty of protein, salmon also helps lower heart disease. Replace beef or other meats with salmon two to three times a week for a leaner, more nutrient-rich protein source.

SHELLFISH

Shellfish may be the most nutritious sea creatures we know of. Clams, oysters, and mussels, among others, rank high on the oceanic food list. Excellent sources of B12 and other vitamins, these foods also contain a ton of zinc, potassium, and iron. Consume sparingly, perhaps on a celebratory night out or during other special occasions.

The foods mentioned above are some of the highest valued foods for IF. Work them into your diet as well as you can, and don't be afraid to get creative with preparation techniques. Keep note of the foods that you already have in your diet and the ones you want to add to your new diet.

CHAPTER 6: TYPES OF INTERMITTENT FASTING DIETS

Now that we have discussed how your body will react to fasting, let's discuss the many different forms of fasting. Although there are seemingly infinite ways to go about your Intermittent Fasting routine, we will focus on six methods that are popular among fitness experts and the fasting community. We will discuss the suitable timing of 'eating windows,' the duration of time in the day when you are allowed to eat, and compare each method so you can successfully choose the best one for your lifestyle. Although fasting has its roots in religion and spirituality, we will not go extensively into these practices, but if you wish to combine your spiritual goals with these methods, you can go right ahead.

At this point, we would like to state that keeping a fasting notebook helps immensely for someone just starting out. By recording our experiences and documenting how successful or unsuccessful our routine is, we can find insight into ourselves and also organize the aspects of our routine that may need to be altered or customized. It is not mandatory to have a notebook, but throughout this book, we will be keeping track of our experiences and analyzing our regimen to understand better what works for us as individuals.

As we move on to explore these popular methods, take note of what they entail and which styles pique your interest as you learn about them. The methods we will explore are as follows:

1. The 16/8 Method

2.   The 5:2 Method

3.   The Eat Stop Eat Method

4.   Alternating Day Fasts

5.   The Warrior Method

6.   The Spontaneity Method

We will also be discussing tips for customizing your routine. The point of this is to personalize your fasting, so it suits you perfectly. This will optimize the results and also allow the practice to become something you created for yourself, which in turn, builds an intimate relationship with your practice promoting dedication and confidence.

The particular method you choose will have a great deal to do with your day-to-day schedule and mindset. Let's choose wisely and give much thought to the various benefits of different methods, but keep in mind the result can be obtained through any of these methods. Let's also be fair in saying that the time windows can be altered to give or take an hour if need be. If one method doesn't quite work for you, do not be disheartened; simply try another method or customize your current choice.

THE 16/8 METHOD

Also known as Leangains method, this method was popularized by Martin Berkhan. The eating window for this style is eight hours with a sixteen-hour fasting time. So if you sleep eight hours, awake, then restrict caloric intake for eight hours, then you can eat as much as you like until bedtime. Another example would be to awake, start your eight-hour eating window, then begin fasting for the evening and during sleep. This is a common choice for people who already skip breakfast. Tea and coffee have no calories, so they are still allowed to be consumed, obviously without sugar added.

Overview:

- Sixteen hours of fasting

- Eight-hour consumption window

- **<u>Zero-calorie drinks allowed</u>**

THE 5/2 DIET METHOD

This method looks more like a diet than a proper fast, but it is a popular method for weight loss and often finds its way into IF circles. First popularized by Michael Mosley, it is also called the 'Fast Diet.' This method involves your normal eating routine for five days of the week, then restricting your caloric intake to 600 calories or less for two days of the week. So you can choose your two days to fast whether they are together or not, let's say Wednesday and Friday. Then, treat all other days like normal days, but on Wednesday and Friday, you eat one or two small meals that together equal 600 calories or less. This is a great beginner diet to try before you get into some more intensive IF. If you're wary of how you may react to fasting, then this method is great to start.

Overview:

- Five days of normal meals according to your daily diet

- **<u>Two days of consuming 600 calories or less</u>**

THE EAT STOP EAT METHOD

This is 24 hours of no solid food or caloric intake. Unsweetened coffee and tea are acceptable during the fasting days for this method. A great example would be to fast from dinner to dinner or, let's say, from 4:00 pm to 4:00 pm the next day. It does not matter what time frame you choose, but it should be a solid 24-hour period. Keeping to your usual eating schedule on the non-fasting days is important.

Overview:

- Strict 24-hour fast once or twice a week

- Maintain usual eating schedule during non-fast days

THE ALTERNATIVE DAY METHOD

This method involves fasting every other day. This method can be customized to your liking on the fast days. You can cut back to 600 calories a day, not unlike the 5/2 method, but fasting every other day. If you feel comfortable, you can intake zero calories on fast days; this would be a very intense method and is not recommended for beginners. For example, eat normally on Sunday, lower calorie intake to 600 calories or less on Monday, eat normally on Tuesday, lower calorie intake Wednesday, eat normally on Thursday, lower calories on Friday. You see, we hit a snag in our pattern as there is an odd number of days in a week. For the odd day out, in this case, Saturday, you can choose to lower the calorie count or eat regularly. It is up to you. For another example, the Saturday odd day out, you could potentially fast for 24 hours then jump back into the pattern on Sunday.

Overview:

- Fast or lower calories every other day

- Keep a usual eating schedule on non-fast days

- **Choose what suits you best for the odd day out**

THE WARRIOR METHOD

This method was popularized by Ori Hofmekler. It includes eating small amounts of raw plant-based foods during the day, then one large meal during the evening. Essentially, you are fasting all day and breaking the fast at night. This diet typically focuses on eating raw and unprocessed foods to get the full benefit. For example, during the day, you snack on fruits, veggies, and nuts. Once the evening comes, you prepare a large meal that is as unprocessed and raw as possible.

Overview:

- Light amounts of raw foods or completely fasting during daylight hours

- **A large meal at night, as unprocessed and raw as possible**

THE SPONTANEITY METHOD

This method is the loosest and most flexible method of IF. The method is pretty straightforward; there are no guidelines or structures. Simply skip a meal when it's convenient or if you're not hungry. Skipping one or two meals every so often can be a great foundation to lay while you search for a more suitable routine. This method also comes in handy for busy people, parents, or just people who love winging it.

Overview:

- No structure

- **Simply skip meals when convenient or fast whenever you like**

CUSTOMIZATION TECHNIQUES

Now that we have a general idea of different fasting techniques, let's keep in mind that these are guidelines that can be customized to fit your specific lifestyle. To reiterate: no one way suits everyone. So as you analyze these methods, keep in mind your personal life and how you alter the structures not only to fit into your schedule but also to personalize your practice. By personalizing your routine, you allow yourself some added empowerment and something that you helped create. Some examples of customizing your practice can include changing the length of fasts, changing diet to suit (vegan, Paleo, etc.), and/or changing the fasting patterns (alternating every two days, etc.).

With the methods above, we see many similarities between them. With the main premise being a caloric restriction and eating window restriction, these methods are simply different customized versions of fasting itself. So this means that we can customize these methods to suit our needs and preferences as individuals.

When we decide to customize a method, it needs to be well thought out. *Why do I need these customizations? Are these customizations feasible as something I can accomplish?* There is an infinite number of ways we can change and alter these techniques, and we will provide some examples below. Keep in mind these are not the only ways to customize, but just some basic strategies. Customize as you please, but be safe and mindful in doing so:

CUSTOMIZATION TECHNIQUE #1: ALTERING THE DURATION OF EATING WINDOWS

We see above that one of the main differences in these methods is the timing. For example, the 16/8 method requires eating for eight hours of the day and fasting for sixteen hours of the day. This can be altered easily to suit you. Need a little extra time for the eating window? Add an hour. Feeling confident that you can shorten the eating window? Shorten it an hour or two. You can also choose your eating window during the day. Morning, midday, or night are all suitable times to eat, depending on your schedule.

CUSTOMIZATION TECHNIQUE #2: ALTERING DAYS

The days in which you choose to fast are very important but not limited to the guidelines above. The alternating method as an example, alternating days of fasting is a simple pattern, but what if you need two days off from fasting? Make your fast days every third day. Another example would be putting more fast days together, as with the Eat Stop Eat method. Instead of one or two days of complete calorie restriction, maybe do three or push your two days back-to-back for a more challenging fast.

CUSTOMIZATION TECHNIQUE #3: ALTERING THE TIMING OF MEALS

Much content online will suggest a proper time for having your meals or will cite the warrior method as an example that requires a large meal at night. This large meal can be placed anywhere in the day according to your preference; in fact, many people prefer their large meal in the middle of the day to avoid a full stomach while sleeping.

CUSTOMIZATION STRATEGY #4: ALTERING MEAL CHOICES

As noted above, the warrior method requires raw foods to be ingested. Many people have dietary restrictions and preferences that may not fit into these diets and methods, so switch it up! What you eat during your IF routines is important, and you want to keep it healthy. But be reasonable with yourself; choose foods you enjoy. If you prefer fried, greasy foods, maybe try the same ingredients but prepared differently – baked chicken instead of breaded and fried, etc.

CUSTOMIZATION STRATEGY #5: INCLUDE YOUR LIFESTYLE

When we research fasting online, we see a pattern – health blogs with muscular people in their fitness attire smiling brightly in front of a sunset. This is all fine for some people, but many do not relate to this lifestyle. Lucky for us, fasting is for everyone. You can add fasting to your normal routine easily without hitting the gym or buying spandex. Make it a point to meld IF into your lifestyle rather than view it as something separate from you. Any hobby you love – gaming, fishing, reading, music, art, scrapbooking, etc. – can be a part of your fasting routine. In fact, having a low-intensity hobby is great for downtime during fasts. Let's not be discouraged if you're not a health nut. Include fasting regardless of your preferred lifestyle, and it will improve it.

These five strategies barely scratch the surface of all the different ways we can alter our routine to fit our lifestyles. Often enough, when we start a fasting routine and get comfortable with the practice, it alters itself naturally to suit our lives. Move with the natural current of things and let your body do the talking. Think deeply about the many strategies available to you and find creative ones to personalize your practice.

We've examined some of the more popular methods of IF and how any method can be altered and customized to fit anyone's needs. While the methods listed above are not the end-all-be-all of IF, they are some of the more popular techniques for a reason. The fitness experts and health gurus that meticulously study and practice these methods present them for the masses online because they work. Another factor being that in our fast-paced society, these methods seem to be some of the better fitting techniques.

CHAPTER 7: DRINKS TO HAVE AND AVOID WHILE INTERMITTENT FASTING

When you go about your first round of intermittent fasting, you'll need to know what to avoid and what to keep close at hand. The following portion of this chapter will reveal exactly what's safe, what to avoid, and what does what for you.

When it comes to foods, the best things to have around are:

- All Legumes and Beans – good carbs can help lower body weight without planned calorie restriction

- Anything high in protein – helpful in keeping your energy levels up in your efforts as a whole, even when you're in a period of fasting

- Anything with the herbs cayenne pepper, psyllium, or dried/crushed dandelion – they'll contribute to weight loss without sacrificing calories or effort

- Avocado – a high-, good-calorie fruit that has a lot of healthy fats

- Berries – often high in antioxidants and vitamin C as well as flavonoids for weight loss

- Cruciferous Vegetables – Broccoli, cauliflower, Brussels sprouts and more are incredibly high in fiber, which you'll definitely want to keep constipation at bay with IF

- Eggs – high in protein and great for building muscle during IF periods

- Nuts & Grains – sources of healthy fats and essential fiber

- Potatoes – when prepared in healthy ways, they satiate hunger well and help with weight loss

- Wild-Caught Fish – high in healthy fats while providing protein and vitamin D for your brain

When it comes to liquids, some of it is pretty self-explanatory:

Water:

- It's always good for you! It will help keep you hydrated, it will provide relief with headaches or lightheadedness, or fatigue, and it clears out your system in the initial detox period.

- Try adding a squeeze of lemon, some cucumber or strawberry slices, or a couple of sprigs of mint, lavender, or basil to give your water some flavor if you're not enthused with the taste of it plain.

If you need something other than water to drink, you can always seek out:

- Probiotic drinks like kefir or kombucha

- You can even look for probiotic foods such as sauerkraut, kimchi, miso, pickles, yogurt, tempeh, and more!

- Probiotics work amazingly well at healing your gut, especially in times of intense transition, as with the start of intermittent fasting.

- Black coffee

- Sweeteners and milk aren't productive for your fasting and weight loss goals.

- Try black coffee whenever possible, in moderation.

- Heated or chilled vegetable or bone broths

- Teas of any kind

- Apple cider vinegar shots

- Instead, try water or other drinks with ACV mixed in.

Drinks to avoid would be:

- Regular soda

- Diet soda

- Alcohol of any kind

- High-sugar coconut and almond drinks

- i.e., coconut water, coconut milk, almond milk, etc.

- Go for the low-sugar or unsweetened milk alternative if it's available.

- Anything with artificial sweetener

- Artificial sweeteners will shock your insulin levels into imbalance with your blood sugar later on.

3 DRINKS TO AVOID

On the flip side, some drinks will definitely push you back from your goals, so keep an eye out for the 3 listed below! Avoid them at all costs.

Sodas of any kind, whether diet or non-diet, are to be avoided absolutely. They are high in sugar and riddled with terrible things for your body. Try to steer clear of this drink, especially during fast periods.

Coconut and almond drinks that are high in sugar are also to be avoided. Artificial sweeteners are killers for one's blood sugar and insulin levels. They will reverse all the good work you've done, so be cautious.

Alcohol will distract you from your focus and commitment to the fast, and it will also steer your body off-course from where you want it to be. Try to IF soberly.

10 GREAT DRINKS

Even when you *are* fasting, drinks are still allowed! Make sure to choose drinks that are nutritious but not too filling, and mix it up whenever you can to keep things from getting stagnant for your taste buds (and body). 10 of the best drinks to incorporate for IF are listed below.

Water with fruit or veggie slices will provide nourishment and flavor for those times when you're fasting and need a little extra boost!

Probiotic drinks like kombucha or kefir will work to heal your gut and tide you over till the next eating window.

Black coffee will become your new best friend, but be sure not to add cream and sugar! They detract from the good work coffee can do for your body during IF.

Teas of any kind are soothing as well as healing for various elements of the body, mind, and soul. Once again, be sure to omit the cream and sugar!

Chilled or heated broths made from vegetables, bone, or animals can sustain one's energy during times of fast, too.

Apple Cider Vinegar shots are great for the tummy and for healing overall! Hippocrates' remedy for any ailment included this and a healthy regimen of fasting occasionally, so you're sure to succeed with this trick.

Water with salt can provide electrolytes, hydration, and brief sustenance for anyone whose stomachs won't stop grumbling.

Fresh-pressed juices are always great for the body, mind, and soul, and in times of IF, they can sustain one's energy and mood during day-long fast periods, in particular.

Wheatgrass shots are just as healthy as ACV shots, with a whole other subset of benefits. To awaken your body and give a jolt to your system, try these on for size.

Coconut water is more hydrating than standard water, and it's full of additional nutrients, too! Try this alternative if you need some enhancement to your usual water.

CHAPTER 8: TIPS AND TRICKS FOR A SMOOTH TRANSITION INTO INTERMITTENT FASTING AND FOR SUCCESSFUL INTERMITTENT FASTING

It can be really daunting to maintain your state of intermittent fasting. One can be tempted by external factors, which can lead that person to quit. However, remember that you started this for a reason. You want to meet that end goal, which is weight loss.

To ensure that you stick to your schedule and fulfill your daily fasting goals, you will need to follow certain tips that will help you overcome the temptations.

Here are some tips:

STAY HYDRATED

Hydration is the key to many things. People usually get some percentage of water from their meals. When you are restricting your eating habits, you are losing your normal water intake. Therefore, you will need to drink lots of water to ensure that your body retains its hydration level throughout the fasting period. As you already know, intermittent fasting allows you to drink water, coffee, tea, or similar beverages even during fasting hours; use this to your advantage by consuming a glass of water every hour.

AVOID BEING TEMPTED BY FOOD

As mentioned earlier, you will have plenty of distractions daily. You will notice people living with you and around you enjoying various delights without worry. You may be tempted to try them every now and then. This is when you are being tested. Overcome it by focusing on the end goal. Think of what you will achieve after you complete your intermittent fasting routine.

RELAX YOUR MIND AND REST A LOT

You will experience a lot of weakness and feel compelled to grab a snack. However, the key to winning during your fasting hours is to relax and rest as much as you can. If you have time, lay down and watch a movie. You can even sleep if you want. Just try to stay away from food and avoid burning calories. Otherwise, you will feel hungrier.

ENSURE THAT EVERY NUTRIENT IS CONSUMED EFFICIENTLY

Intermittent fasting will also challenge your body in terms of nutrients. You will have to ensure that you are consuming all your necessary nutrients. This will give you the energy you need for the day. Choose foods that are rich in healthy fats, fiber, and protein. You can even consume fat-soluble vitamin supplements to keep your body healthy. Research properly and invest your time and effort in meals that will be highly beneficial for you during your IF routine.

Furthermore, choosing foods that are high in nutrients after your fasting period can control your blood sugar levels as well as balance the nutrients in your body. Any deficiency could result in medical conditions. You don't want that to happen, do you?

CONSUME FOODS HIGH IN VOLUME BUT LOW IN CALORIES

This is also important so that you have a filling meal. However, make sure that the food you are choosing is not high in calories. You can choose foods like fruits, raw vegetables, popcorn, etc. These can be eaten in a quantity that creates a full meal. Plus, you should choose foods that have high moisture content.

CONSUME LOW-CALORIE FOODS THAT TASTE GOOD

Sometimes the body doesn't crave more food; rather, it craves certain flavors. These flavors can be easily found in various items such as vinegar, spices, herbs, garlic, etc. You may simply be needing these flavors in your meal. Plus, these items are low in calories. Eating them in your meal will help suppress hunger.

Intermittent fasting may not have a strict schedule, but it does have some aftereffects that must be dealt with. With dedication and commitment, you can overcome them and achieve your desired healthful results.

CHAPTER 9: WHO CAN DO INTERMITTENT FASTING AND WHO CANNOT

The following pages will address five different profiles of candidates who wouldn't be conducive to growing and healing with the intermittent fasting meal plan. Of course, the sex distinction in our studies of intermittent fasting plays a huge role in this chapter, for the intersections of sex and disease or disorder are what makes these candidates so problematic about IF itself. From the pregnant candidate to the underweight woman, the female patient with the eating disorder, the female diabetic, and the woman with the troubling personality, it remains true that intermittent fasting isn't necessarily for everyone.

However, even with these limitations in place, there is lingering potential for each of these types of women to come to a place of progress or healing eventually that would allow them to move through their struggles and attempt IF at their own pace. Therefore, if you qualify as any of the following candidates, don't be too dejected or hopeless! With the appropriate personal growth and the right lessons being presented to you, you'll surely come back to intermittent fasting as soon as you're ready for it.

EXPLORING THE PREGNANT CANDIDATE

Although intermittent fasting can give you increased energy, better metabolism, and stronger cellular protection, the risks clearly outweigh the benefits for pregnant IF candidates. Since the female body is made to bear children, the effects of intermittent fasting are already debated in their relation to female health, but when it comes to pregnant and soon-to-be mothers, the answer to the question is a clear "No." Pregnant women should not be working with intermittent fasting.

For the expecting mother, long periods between meals are not necessarily such a good thing. The pregnant woman will need to be eating whenever she's hungry to gain the weight and nutrients her future child will need to survive. Furthermore, she will need to combat the morning sickness and nausea that go along with pregnancy, and if she's concerned about her timing with the intermittent fast, she might put herself in a detrimental situation for her overall health by mistake.

If you're recently pregnant but had used intermittent fasting previously with great success, you can shift back to focusing on what you eat rather than when you eat. Just as it is for the standard person shifting from normal eating to intermittent fasting and going from what's eaten to when it's eaten, when you switch from IF to pregnancy, you'll shift eating habits once again. This time, however, you'll try to make sure you're eating the best foods whenever possible, not just in your okayed eating windows.

If you're having trouble stopping your intermittent fast while you've just become pregnant, you might want to reconsider the reasons behind your IF in the first place. Is it really for your health, or does it support your controlling tendency to limit your weight? Try to make sure that when you're pregnant, you're looking for what supports your health, rather than your mental image of what you should look like and what you think you should weigh. Pregnancy is a beautiful time, but it's not about restriction, it's about abundance and weight gain and growth, so it doesn't mesh well with IF at all.

EXPLORING THE UNDERWEIGHT CANDIDATE

For women who are already underweight, intermittent fasting might not be the best thing for your health. Surely, there are unintentionally underweight women who don't have the time they'd like to have for eating or who don't have the energy they'd like to have for cooking, but there are also intentionally underweight women who are looking for an additional method to use to keep off that "excess" weight for good.

If you're incredibly underweight already (even if you don't feel like it!), steer clear of intermittent fasting. If you're only five to ten pounds underweight and you're seeking spiritual enlightenment, lessened brain fog, or a jolt to your digestive system, IF may work just fine for you without being problematic. (While you might find a method of IF that works alright for you in this case, don't make the hard and fast decisions on eating pattern switching without first making sure to consult a doctor or health professional.)

Essentially, the problem arises when the individual is already over 10 pounds underweight, for these individuals aren't giving their digestive systems a break or a free moment for healing by switching to IF. Instead, the individual in this stance forces his or her digestive system to claw at itself and scrape at the bottom of the barrel to try and heal itself. I shouldn't have to explain why that simply won't work.

Overall, something you can use to determine whether you're in the healthy or unhealthy weight range is your BMI (Body Mass Index). If your BMI is anywhere between 18.5 and 25, you're in the healthy weight range. However, if you're lower than 18.5, be cautious about attempting intermittent fasting. If you're lower than 17, definitely do **not** try this method, for your body can't stand to lose anything else, and to choose IF would cause extreme detriment to your health rather than aid it.

EXPLORING THE CANDIDATE WITH AN EATING DISORDER

For the individual with an eating disorder, no matter what variety, intermittent fasting may seem to be helpful, but it will only function as a trigger for that person's disorder. No matter who you are, if you approach intermittent fasting for healing or weight loss, you're probably doing so because you want to switch from stuffing yourself with emptiness to healing yourself with goodness. Your focus, in other words, likely falls on growth (not physically but emotionally, spiritually, mentally, and regarding health capacity) rather than withering.

For the individual suffering from an eating disorder, all attempts toward health and growth are skewed by distortions of body image and self-esteem. Essentially, all attempts toward health and growth are twisted by the compulsory drive to purge. If you or someone you know struggled or struggles with anorexia, bulimia, orthorexia, binge eating, purging, avoidant/restrictive food intake disorder, or any other eating disorder, be extremely curious and demanding with them if they share an interest in intermittent fasting.

Question their inspirations and drives; demand they are honest with you. The likelihood is greater than not that this person is using intermittent fasting as a way to lose weight that they can't afford to lose rather than to get healthier in general. If you're able to discern it at all, the individual's reason for starting IF is the best way to ascertain their true intentions. It can be hard to tell who has an eating disorder and who doesn't, but the way people talk about food, body image, fasting, and dieting can reveal more than you could ever anticipate. And once you **can** tell who has an eating disorder, help them stay clear from IF because it can really exacerbate their circumstances despite their (and your) best intentions.

EXPLORING THE DIABETIC CANDIDATE

If you're already on insulin, as a diabetic, most likely, you're already working to keep your levels of blood sugar at balance. If you add into the mix IF work to increase or decrease insulin resistance (to help with weight loss), you'll put yourself in a truly dangerous spot. People with diabetes should absolutely not skip doses of insulin to lose weight by lowering blood sugar. This would be disastrous for someone who has diabetes because they'd surely lose the weight, but they'd feel drained to a disastrous degree because humans do need this sugar or glucose in our blood to derive energy.

So, if you have diabetes, stay away from intermittent fasting. It's unfortunate, I know, but this type of eating pattern change will do absolutely nothing good for you. As with the pregnant candidate, you could try to switch the foods you're eating instead of when you're eating. By adding the right, healthful foods into your diet, you might find that the weight that sticks to you so stubbornly can be depleted with your condition being made none the worse. However, be careful if you're diabetic when it comes to fasting disguised as dieting. If you feel inclined to try a juice or liquid diet, guess those inclinations, for it's very likely that this type of diet would cause extra stress to your system, what with the high glycemic and fiber-free contents of some juices.

Basically, if you're diabetic and feeling inclined to make your life healthier, don't limit when you eat and don't just drink liquids. Rather than restricting whatsoever, try to incorporate healthier, more whole foods that are oriented towards healing innately, and then maybe add exercise into the mix when you're ready for it.

EXPLORING PROBLEMATIC CHARACTER TRAITS

While the previous entries in this chapter have to deal with physical traits and conditions, this final one has to do more so with personality and character attributes instead. The truth of the matter is that some personality types will not mesh well with the lifestyle connected to intermittent fasting. Whether you're controlling, OCD, impatient, moody, reserved, or just too young, you're not in for a "treat" by taking the first steps toward the intermittent fasting lifestyle. Nevertheless, the fact holds that if you can work through your struggles and face your (personality) demons, you might find yourself changed by intermittent fasting in ways no one would have ever expected.

Controlling people expect the world to be easily manipulated to suit their needs, urges, and comforts. Unfortunately, the world doesn't often act so easily shapeable, which puts controlling individuals in tough places. In fasting and dieting especially, control goes out the window, and natural progress/timelines take their place. Therefore, controlling individuals might have trouble adjusting to intermittent fasting. Although these people will be able to make changes to their techniques as they go along, they still won't be able to actualize the changes they want with any immediacy. For controlling people, working with intermittent fasting will be a huge challenge, but it's definitely not impossible.

People who are impatient will also have a hard time with intermittent fasting because of what their expectations of the world happen to be. Impatient people expect the world to go fast, for things to be where they expect it when they expect it, and for progress to be made when they're ready for it to be made. In essence, impatient people are the opposite of productive intermittent fasters, for people skilled and practiced with IF know that patience is the ultimate virtue. It takes two weeks only to get fully past just the detoxification period for intermittent fasting, so clearly, impatient people will need those urges recalibrated before they're ready to handle the personal practice of consistency and waiting that gives life to the IF technique (and lifestyle).

Moody individuals will likely only see their emotional situations worsened by intermittent fasting, but these types of people often don't choose to fast intermittently because they want to fix their mood disorders. Instead, these people choose IF to lose weight, gain energy, fight aging and heal themselves, and the emotional side-effects are just that. I recommend these individuals look at the bigger picture of intermittent fasting. This eating pattern and lifestyle change can make great waves in one's life that cause him or her to feel increasingly moody or troubled. By having increased awareness of the bigger picture, moody people might be able to hold off on transitioning to IF until they're healed enough to handle all the switch has to offer.

People who are excessively reserved or conservative in personality may find that intermittent fasting doesn't work for them because they struggle through the detox period and can't get any farther. It is true that the first two weeks of intermittent fasting – the detox period – are intense, both physically and emotionally. Sometimes, people break down into tears or have emotional explosions otherwise during this detoxification time, and overly reserved or conservative individuals will likely **not** appreciate being exposed to moments like this, much less that potential within their selves. If these types of people can learn to laugh at themselves and ride emotional waves more calmly, they'll have as much to gain from IF as any of the best of us.

Finally, when considering young people under the age of 18, we get back into physical traits and conditions a bit more than character traits, but it's undeniable that someone's youth makes it very difficult for intermittent fasting to work in his or her favor. No offense, but you're immature, and your body is even more immature, so you need all the available nutrients around you to help you grow properly. Limiting nutritional intake in any way (whether it's the what you eat or when it happens) will not be good for you until you're at least 18 and living your best life in that strong, fully-actualized, adult body.

CHAPTER 10: COMMON MISTAKES

Intermittent fasting supporters believe that this routine can be great for weight loss and increasing mood and energy levels. However, this can be achieved only if one is likely to follow it correctly. If you are going to limit your time and avoid eating, you will need to adjust your daily plan.

While your eating habits remain the same, your schedule changes drastically, as you are skipping regular meals. You may not even realize that you are not doing it correctly. That is why this section will focus on certain errors that IF followers sometimes do not realize they are making while on the diet schedule.

Review the mistakes and remember to avoid them at all costs.

CHANGING YOUR DIET CONSIDERABLY

When you are planning to change your diet to suit your fasting schedule for the first time, you are supposed to take it slow. Some think that they are strong enough to bear the pressure of fasting for multiple hours on their first go. However, they soon realize that their bodies are unable to handle the sudden drastic change.

Instead of acting tough, it is better to switch to the fasting cycle progressively. Taking it slow and steady will give you the best results. So, avoid the mistake of fasting for eight full hours and that, too, during non-sleeping hours. This can lead to negative effects on the body.

EATING IN EXCESS WHEN YOUR FASTING PERIOD ENDS

This situation can be counterproductive. If you fast religiously and then fill your stomach with excessive food, what is the use of such a diet plan in the first place? Overeating will simply bring back all the calories you worked so hard to lose. Don't overeat.

Instead, plan the right way of dealing with this situation. If possible, prepare a set of meals that you are going to consume during your intermittent fasting days. Choosing healthy and limited options will give you a better way of dealing with hunger. Plus, you can choose healthy options that will give you the strength you are going to need.

CONSUMING LIQUIDS THAT YOU SHOULD NOT BE DRINKING

IF gives you the freedom to consume liquids, but that does not mean you are free to consume all beverages. Your choices of drinks should not include too many calories or too much sugar, nor should you consume sodas or alcohol. The maximum you can do is add a packet of stevia (but do not overuse it) or some milk to your coffee or tea. Choosing such ingredients will ensure that you have a better chance of being prepared for your fasting period.

Another thing to note is that you should not consume liquids that are filled with proteins, like bone broth. Liquids with high protein content can stop the process of autophagy. (This process helps with cell repair.) You do not want to stop this process that you worked so hard to achieve through your intermittent fasting technique.

To fix this error, focus on improving your hydration. Stick to water as much as possible for best results.

CHOOSING UNHEALTHY FOODS

People who practice intermittent fasting tend to lose nutrients unless they focus on the quality of foods consumed. Anyone can easily feel like rewarding himself or herself for working hard to avoid delicious treats during fasting hours. Later, he or she may think about consuming something unhealthy during eating hours. This mistake can lead to an unbalanced diet that will eliminate all the health benefits achieved so far.

You can fix this by monitoring your eating schedule. Keep track of what you are eating during your eating hours. If you still crave certain flavors, be sure to choose healthy meals.

Remember that mistakes can be avoided if you are aware of them. Focus on preplanning everything so you do not have to decide spontaneously. That will benefit you the most and give you the upper hand at maintaining your intermittent schedule for a longer period.

CHAPTER 11: DOES INTERMITTENT FASTING HAVE DIFFERENT EFFECTS ON MEN AND WOMEN?

INTERMITTENT FASTING AND FEMALE FERTILITY

Because health, diet, reproductivity, and nutritional needs are all altered for mature and menopausal women, their relationships with intermittent fasting can be very different from young women's. For instance, while young women ought to be careful about how intermittent fasting can affect their fertility levels, older women can practice intermittent fasting freely without these concerns. Therefore, more mature women can apply the weight-loss techniques of intermittent fasting to their lives (and waistlines) without worrying about what negative side-effects might arise in the future.

For menopausal women, however, the situation is a little bit different from that of fully mature women. People going through menopause have to deal with daily hormone fluctuations that cause hot and cold flashes, sleeplessness, anxiety, irregular periods, and more. At the beginning of this process, intermittent fasting will not necessarily help, and it could even make your situation more stressful.

For women in this situation who are actively going through menopause, you must remember that your body is extremely sensitive to changes right now. If you do find that intermittent fasting helps and that short periods of fast are effective, you must also make sure to increase the intensity of your fast as gradually as possible so your body can adjust without creating horrible hormonal repercussions for yourself and everyone around you.

For the fully mature woman, intermittent fasting will not make you as cranky, moody, and irregular in the period, or otherwise because those hormones won't be affecting you at all anymore, or at least, hardly at all. Your dietary and eating schedule choices become more liberated from the effects they used to have on your hormonal health as the years go by. Therefore, if you're seeking weight loss, better energy, a physiological jolt back to health, or what have you, try out IF without concern and see what happens. For these types of women, intermittent fasting is set to provide hope through eased depression, the lessened likelihood of cancer (or its recurrence), promised weight loss, and more.

INTERMITTENT FASTING DURING MENSTRUATION

Another subset of women that should be cautious when approaching intermittent fasting is those who struggle with PCOS. This acronym stands for a hormonal disorder called Polycystic Ovary Syndrome that causes the woman's reproductive system to dysfunction in certain ways that lead to pain, weight gain, missed periods, and hormonal imbalances of a variety of kinds.

While some people believe women with PCOS shouldn't overly stress their systems with something like intermittent fasting, others think that IF is exactly what these ladies need. In this chapter, we'll go over the details of PCOS as well as how intermittent fasting can actually help. Furthermore, we'll approach dietary tips, treatments, and exercises for women with this condition, and we'll end with the best IF-inspired ways for these women to lose weight.

By the end of this chapter, you should have a hunch whether or not you have PCOS, and if you already know that you have it, you should feel confident about whether or not intermittent fasting can help you. Regardless of what path you choose, the final three sections of this chapter should provide you with somewhat of a cheat-sheet to interact with the world on a more health-oriented level, whether through food, treatment, exercise, or weight loss.

WHAT IS PCOS?

For women with PCOS, life can be miserable. Periods can be unpredictable, and these women's bodies can become almost like foreign worlds, what with all the hormones going haywire. Essentially, PCOS is a hormonal imbalance that affects the reproductive health and metabolism Of those who live out the condition. This imbalance of reproductive hormones causes issues for these women's ovaries, causing them to have trouble releasing eggs as they should.

Although the name of the disorder speaks of cysts, many women do not develop cysts on their ovaries with this condition. Instead, all women with PCOS develop pools of excess fluids in their ovaries, they produce a surplus of androgens (commonly known as "male hormones"), they're all less responsive to insulin, and they all experience a relative lack of progesterone (which contributes more to those irregular periods).

The overall symptoms of PCOS are extra hair growth or early balding (caused by that androgen!), acne, headaches, mood swings, fatigue, weight gain, insomnia or light sleep, pelvic pain, and even infertility. Therefore, this disorder can make women extra cranky, heavy, sleepy, sad, and bald. It's not a fun fight! When it comes to PCOS, however, there are a couple of things you can try, and one of them is – you guessed it! – intermittent fasting.

BEST TREATMENTS & EXERCISES FOR PCOS

Whether you want to combine PCOS with intermittent fasting or not, there are a few other treatments and exercises to consider to mitigate the effects of your condition. After trying out a few of these, if things still haven't gotten better, maybe a more drastic measure such as intermittent fasting will help you more. It's hard to say for sure at this moment, but as always, move forward with your doctor's approval to ensure your path to health is the best one for the situation.

As far as treatments go, there are a few directions you can go. There are (1) medicinal treatments, (2) alleviation of symptom treatments, and (3) lifestyle treatments. In terms of medicinal treatments, you could try using a birth control method (i.e., the pill, the patch, the shot, an IUD, or the vaginal ring) that works primarily on hormones. This will help regulate your period, lower cancer risk, and help with acne and hair issues. You could also try medicines that block androgens in your body to get rid of that acne and hair loss. These pills are often problematic if you want to become pregnant in the future, though. Additionally, you could try Metformin (used to treat type 2 diabetes, but helps with PCOS symptoms too); Provera (regulates menses through providing progesterone); Clomiphene/Clomid, Letrozole/Femara, or Gonadotropins (medications that help increase and regulate ovulation); Eflornithine or Electrolysis (to help with slowing facial hair growth, if necessary); or Progestin therapy (protects against cancer and regulates periods, but won't help with androgen). Many of these medical treatments are treatments that tie into symptom-alleviation as well.

The third option is lifestyle treatments, whereby bigger decisions and life changes are meant to help the individual heal and cope with their disorder. In this case, fasting, IF, or dieting are great additions along with exercise. If and when you decide to incorporate exercise into your lifestyle (to help heal or otherwise), you can make sure your workouts include one or more of these five tactics so that you're getting the most out of the experience (in ways that benefit your condition, too).

First, go for some cardio. Cardio training has the ability to increase mood, stabilize fertility, and help with your insulin resistance issue. Whether it's walking, jogging, cycling, swimming, or otherwise, even just 30 minutes a day of cardio works wonders on your weight while helping with other side-effects of PCOS. If you do nothing else, incorporate cardio into your daily routine, and you'll already be feeling better in no time.

Second, try strength training! Equally helpful for your insulin resistance issue, strength training like cardio improves insulin function in the body while boosting metabolism and contributing to good moods.

Third, if you've never heard of the pelvic floor, you're in for a "treat"! You can always use pelvic floor strengthening to lessen that pelvic pain and tension that you might feel on a daily basis. You don't even need to go to the gym to do this. All you have to do is squeeze your butt-cheeks together. You'll feel that, nearer to your vulva, you have another squeezing occurring, too. See if you can isolate that sensation. As you get better at doing exactly that, you'll become able to squeeze for five breaths and release. The longer you can complete these repetitions of squeezing and releasing, the stronger your pelvic floor will be! There are also tools you can find in certain stores and online that are oriented towards pelvic floor strengthening when you get to that point.

Fourth, work on that core strength! Core strength not only makes your body stronger, but it also helps increase senses of well-being and personal power. When your core is strong, you have a much easier time knowing what you want, speaking out about it, and saying "no" when you need to. Just like pelvic floor strengthening, working on core strength will be hugely beneficial when/if you decide to become pregnant.

Fifth, if you're feeling up to it, try HIIT. High-Intensity Interval Training can help you lose 5-10% of your original weight, which is always going to help mitigate PCOS symptoms. The more weight you lose, the less androgen and testosterone are stocked up in your body, and the better insulin resistance you develop.

BEST (IF) TIPS ON HOW TO LOSE WEIGHT FOR PCOS

Overall, losing weight with PCOS is a great goal. Losing weight can help your symptoms become lessened in many ways. It can help your body remember how to regulate insulin; it can help your hormones go back to normal levels; it can help provide daily activity; it can make your body healthier and stronger; and if you want to get pregnant despite your condition, losing weight is an essential step to recover your fertility. A few tips to lose weight through intermittent fasting and otherwise are listed below.

Try out the crescendo method! If you do decide to explicitly incorporate intermittent fasting into your routine as someone with PCOS, go with the crescendo method. Start with just one or two days on a 14:14 fast, and then if the first week feels good on all levels, you might consider trying those one or two days on 16:8 instead or switching to three days at 14:14. The crescendo method is built to be flexible, so try it out and then see if your body wants (and allows) you to stick with it.

Delay your breakfast! You can still try to get that 12-hour, 14-hour, or even 16-hour fast in the right at the beginning of your day by just waiting a little longer for breakfast.

Eat dinner earlier! If you really want to incorporate IF into your PCOS life, try eating dinner earlier to begin your fast each night. You'll easily be able to get 12 or 14 of fast in daily with that adjustment.

Cut out those snacks! You might not be able to try fasting windows each day, and it could be the case that you do try them, and it doesn't make anything better. Instead, try cutting down on your daily snack intake! That simple dietary switch can help enact IF goals in your life as well as its side-effects.

Eat healthier meals! Instead of fasting or exercising intensely, you could always switch to eating healthier meals when you decide it's time to eat. There are some women with PCOS who only have to make this slight adjustment to see the weight loss goals they desire.

Reconsider serving sizes! This point goes hand-in-hand with the one before it. If you redesign your meals to be healthier, whether in content or serving size, you may be able to see your weight loss goals actualized without intermittent fasting whatsoever.

Mesh exercise with dietary change! Since you might decide not to engage with intermittent fasting, given your condition, just be reminded that you can always combine exercise routine and dietary change to achieve the same effects. While women who intermittently fast are often discouraged from incorporating both intense exercise and dietary change into their routine while practicing IF, you don't have to worry about that goal-clash as much.

INTERMITTENT FASTING: PREGNANCY AND BREASTFEEDING

One of the most heated debates in the field of intermittent fasting for women is whether or not it's productive for breastfeeding mothers to engage in intermittent fasting after their babies are born. People tend to feel strongly about their opinions in this debate, but it still comes down to what feels right for you.

If you're skimming through this section as someone who will have babies in the future, just let the ideas settle in and simmer. If you're reading through this book as a pregnant woman, read through these ideas but be sure to ask your doctor before you fully settle either way and make sure to do your rounds of research based on your body type and needs.

This chapter will be dedicated to hashing out the arguments in the field, and it will settle in a neutral stance that both reveals the dangers and the methods that have worked for breastfeeding IF mothers. Ultimately, the chapter will culminate in two sections about diet, the first informing about the standards for eating right while breastfeeding and the second providing five recipes to use in your personal life for health while breastfeeding.

By the end of this section, you should still be a little curious. You might have settled on whether or not you think breastfeeding while intermittent fasting is healthy, but you are likely still questioning. That's great, if so! Take those questions to the internet, to encyclopedias, or your doctor and do the hard work to find out what's right for you. Your body and your baby will be forever thankful you did.

THE ARGUMENTS IN THE FIELD: A GOOD IDEA OR NOT?

When it comes down to the arguments in the field, there are two main camps. Some people think it's fine for mothers to intermittently fast while they're breastfeeding as long as they're following the right guidelines. Other people think it would be abhorrent for a mother even to consider intermittent fasting while she's breastfeeding. Of course, with there being two camps, these ideas demonstrate extremes along a binary, and the best method with extremes of this nature is finding their balance. Therefore, let your balance be established within this ongoing debate, and use the information provided to make the best decision for yourself, your body, and your baby.

In the "Yes" camp of individuals who think you can balance breastfeeding and intermittent fasting, the main argument is that it's only an intermittent fast! This group of individuals tends to think that, of course, a woman can balance breastfeeding and intermittent fasting mostly because every woman, every pregnancy, and every case is different, so of course, every woman would consult her doctor to check and make sure things were okay before actually moving forward with the decision. These people also consider that you should compare your pregnancy goals to your personal goals, and if you'd rather focus on the latter, you may not need to breastfeed whatsoever! The arguments then fragment out from this group's main ideas into themes such as "Yes, IF and breastfeeding can be balanced if it's a short fast," "...if it's a less intense fast," or "...if it's a different diet to compensate." Regardless, the point is the same; you absolutely can plan an intermittent fast that doesn't interfere too much with your breastfeeding or your baby's health.

In the "No" camp of individuals who think you should never try to balance breastfeeding and intermittent fasting, the main argument is that you're removing your abilities to produce milk, which are so essential for the child and its growth overall. These people see that fewer nutrients will be contained in the milk when the mother consumes fewer nutrients, and they know that milk production itself can decrease when mothers restrict caloric intake. Furthermore, these individuals think that you shouldn't force things (by intermittent fasting) and that you should just ride with nature's punches until breastfeeding is over. It's just six months of waiting, after all, they say. These individuals would ask the breastfeeding mother to consider her intentions when she chooses to restrict food intake during this time. If her goals are motivated by others' opinions, whether of beauty, of what's "natural," or of timing, she is encouraged to question what she actually wants for herself and the baby, what's actually healthy, and what she's doing rushing things in the first place.

POSSIBLE DANGERS

The possible dangers of combining intermittent fasting with breastfeeding are as follows:

LESS MILK! NO MILK!

Yes, the breastfeeding mother will produce less milk when she restricts her caloric intake. This issue can be helped by fasting incredibly rarely and with lowered fast hours, less exercise, and less intensity of food restriction during eating periods. This danger is only legitimate for the mother who truly wants to breastfeed her child consistently as the child's only source of food.

NO ENERGY!

Yes, the breastfeeding mother will have less energy for herself and to pay close attention to her baby if she's restricting caloric intake through intermittent fasting and still able to breastfeed her child for every meal. As long as the mother has a capable and non-disabled partner willing to pick up the slack and pay close attention to everything else, this might still be okay. Frequent check-ups to the doctor will ensure that this low energy level isn't detrimental to mama and baby's health.

IF YOU'RE SICK, IT WILL ONLY MAKE THINGS WORSE!

Yes, it is true that if the breastfeeding mother is sick on top of everything else, intermittent fasting will exacerbate the problem to a dangerous degree for both mama and baby. In these cases, the mother should completely cease intermittent fasting until the sickness is gone. If she continues, her health and her baby's life are at risk.

OTHER CONCERNS: ANEMIA, LOW BLOOD PRESSURE OR SUGAR, ETC

Sometimes, the pregnant mother might have health problems that are made worse through pregnancy and strained even further through the process of intermittent fasting. This reality is the primary reason why you should always check with your doctor before you choose to breastfeed and intermittently fast at the same time. Only your doctor knows all your tics and diseases, so only she will be able to make sure you're making the best choice for yourself and your family.

WHAT METHODS HAVE WORKED

The methods that have worked to combine and balance intermittent fasting with breastfeeding are as follows:

LOW-INTENSITY CRESCENDO METHOD

Because the crescendo method begins with just a few days a week, and those days aren't even full fast days, breastfeeding mothers might be able to work from this starting place to see if things are going to work out with IF at this time or not. If three days a week of basically 16:8 method, then go down to two days. If two days are still too much, go down to one day. If one day then feels good, stay there. If you feel like you can do more, try upping the ante to two days or going back to three days at 14:10 or 12:12 instead. There are ways to make this work!

FLEXIBLE, SPONTANEOUS MEAL SKIPPING

The breastfeeding mother can work with intermittent fasting as long as the plan isn't too structured and restrictive. The most productive method for the woman in this position will be a very flexible, spontaneous skip method. Whenever the mother has fully fed her child and feels lingering energy, she might try skipping her next meal. She might try skipping breakfast daily or cutting out a snack or two. Non-severe restrictions of this nature can be beneficial to both mama and baby, but they do have to be entirely **non-severe**.

ONE WEEK OUT OF THE MONTH

One other method mama can try is to "fast" only one week each month. Maybe she can try going throughout the month as it begins and waits until the last week of the month to see if she feels well and strong enough to produce milk and maintain an intermittent fast. In these cases, the best fasting strategy for that one week might be alternate-day or 5:2. However, 14:10 or 12:12 in that week might work just as well, if not better, for a breastfeeding mom. As always, see what works best for you with slow and flexible experimentation to start.

Another method that can work is, with lack of a better name idea, the "Eventually…" method, whereby the breastfeeding mother realizes that she can intermittently fast once the child is six months old. Some scholars really think that the baby should have mother's milk for the first six months, but that afterward, it doesn't matter so much. Moms can easily piggyback on this logic by riding out the first six months with the baby and then switching to start balancing intermittent fasting with breastfeeding when that time is up, and the need to have breastmilk is lessened for the newborn.

OVERALL TIPS

Overall, if you do decide to intermittently fast while breastfeeding, keep these five tips in mind. First, hydrate! Hydrate to an excessive degree almost, but make sure you're getting a good mix of water, electrolytes, teas, and more. Just water all the time will make you feel faint, dizzy, or lightheaded, none of which are productive whatsoever.

Second, take supplements! Breastfeeding mothers should be getting a variety of nutrients through several sources. If you're intermittent fasting while breastfeeding, one thing you can do to troubleshoot is to take supplements to replace what's being missed or overlooked. Supplements of great necessity are vitamins B1, B2, B6, and B12, choline, vitamins A & D, selenium, iodine, folate, calcium, iron, copper, and zinc.

Third, you don't have to lose that baby weight intermittently fast! Try exercising consistently instead. Try dieting instead. You don't have to stop eating or engage in a pattern like that to lose weight. There are several other things and practices to try to shed post-partum weight. Don't think that IF is the only option, and remember, you can always come back to IF in six months when the baby is older.

Fourth, you can try out intermittent fasting and breastfeeding and use your baby's diaper evidence to see if it's healthy for the child or not. Is the baby's stool runny? It should be! If it becomes solid, you're not getting enough liquids through your body. If it's an abnormal color, something might be up. Check with your doctor if your child's waste looks anything other than normal, for it might be a clue that your intermittent fasting isn't helping at all but rather hurting.

Fifth, no matter what you've decided for your intermittent fast at this time, if you feel or notice any of those warning signs or worst-case-scenario markers, eat something. Your goals to fast are not more important than your baby's and your health. Remember that you're a mother as well as an individual; now more than ever, it's important not to push yourself past the breaking point.

EATING RIGHT WHILE BREASTFEEDING

Making sure you get the right nutrients for your baby while you're breastfeeding, especially IF breastfeeding, is essential! This section will go through facts about different foods and drinks that will be beneficial to your health and the baby's as you attempt breastfeeding, with or without the addition of intermittent fasting. You will learn how to eat smart to help with postpartum weight loss, how to behave in ways that help you lose weight, how to eat without affecting your milk supply, and more.

Avocados are high in healthy fats as well as vitamins B, K, C, & E. Furthermore, avocados are high in potassium and folates that help the breastfeeding mother produce more milk while keeping her body and heart healthy.

Beans & Legumes provide vitamins, minerals, phytoestrogens, and protein! They're great for breastfeeding mothers, especially when a variety of beans and legumes are eaten, for they enable the mother to produce a constantly healthy milk supply.

Blueberries have lots of vitamins and minerals that keep your energy level high through their complex carbohydrates. They're also high in antioxidants to keep you healthy and glowing for your baby!

Brown Rice is a great addition to your diet while breastfeeding, for it grants the calories needed, and it's known to make good-quality milk for babies. These healthy carbs are just what you need.

Eggs, being high in protein, provide fatty acids for your milk and energy for yourself.

Fish like salmon is high in a healthy fat called DHA as well as being low in mercury. If you're looking for protein, healthy fats, omega-3s, and low toxicity, fish is a great place to start.

Fresh or Dried Fruit is always great for breastfeeding mothers! Eat the rainbow every day for the proper nutrients, vitamins, and minerals to regain strength and share it with your baby.

Fresh Vegetables (with Hummus!) is always great for breastfeeding mothers! Eat the rainbow every day for the proper nutrients, vitamins, and minerals to regain strength and share it with your baby.

Leafy Greens are high in magnesium for muscle and joint pain as well as fiber for healthy waste removal from your body (the last thing you want right now is to be constipated!). They also provide an incredible number of minerals for health in general, including vitamins A & C, calcium, and antioxidants.

Lean Beef boosts mama's energy with iron, protein, and vitamin B12, all of which are essential for her energy to be able to keep up with the baby.

Low-Fat Dairy Products such as milk, yogurt, or cheese provide vitamin D, calcium, protein, and more, all of which are essential for building strong bones and developing a baby's immune system.

Mushrooms are thought to contain a lactogenic agent present in both barley and oats that help mothers produce milk for their newborns. The best mushrooms for the job are oyster, maitake, shimeji, shiitake or reishi.

Nuts have so much going on that they should be part of the breastfeeding mother's daily diet. Nuts are high in zinc, calcium, iron, and vitamins K & B. They're also lactogenic, especially almonds, and they provide protein and fatty acids for the mama in these times of need, too.

Oranges give a great energy boost through their vitamin C content.

Red & Orange Root Veggies have been used for their lactogenic potential in many cultures around the world for generations. In particular, carrots and yams are favored when it comes to using food to increase breastfeeding capacity.

Seeds (esp. Chia, Flax, & Hemp) in general are high in protein, calcium, iron, and zinc, but specifically, chia, flax, and hemp seeds are overloaded in omega-3 content. How perfect for a breastfeeding mom!

Starchy Foods (i.e., bread, potatoes, pasta, and rice) provide an excellent source of energy for breastfeeding mothers. If you're intermittently fasting, be sure to include lots of these (balanced with healthy fats!) in your diet.

Turmeric, Fennel, Fenugreek, & Ashwagandha are all incredibly healing herbs that should be used in the cooking of all breastfeeding mothers. The first three are lactogenic, helping breastfeeding mothers produce milk, while the final one is a reproductive, glandular, immune, and neurological booster. It relieves stress, fights disease, and increases the quality of life for everyone who uses it.

Whole Wheat and Grains such as barley and oats are packed with lactogenic potential. They are essential for the breastfeeding mother's diet, especially if she's intermittently fasting.

INTERMITTENT FASTING AND MENOPAUSE

While the greatest concerns about intermittent fasting's effects on women often center on potential problems with reproduction and fertility, some women simply don't have to worry about that anymore. For mature and menopausal women, intermittent fasting poses a different instance and option entirely.

This chapter will be dedicated to the experiences of these women. It will discuss what happens when women age, how their needs change, and how nutrition is affected. Furthermore, it will discuss how intermittent fasting affects both mature and menopausal women before giving suggestions of how to approach IF for each type of woman.

Next, we will walk through some anti-aging foods, tips, and exercises to lose that weight, and then we'll end with the best intermittent fasting method for you at this time. By the time this chapter ends, you should feel confident (as a mature or menopausal woman) that you can approach intermittent fasting safely and productively, and you should have a solid plan in mind regarding how you'll go about that when you're ready.

DIFFERENCES BETWEEN THE YOUNG VS. OLDER WOMAN

At the most basic level, it must be said that there are detailed bodily differences between young women and older women. Many of these bodily differences become obvious with the outward physical effects of aging, but a lot of them also happen on the inside, away from what our eyes can see.

When women age, enter and exit menopause, and become fully mature, their bodies change, reflecting different nutritional needs for the next 30+ years. During menopause, in particular, certain foods help with the urges, hot flashes, and more, but the period of intense transition is more of a gateway into a completely altered future (mentally, bodily, nutritionally, and more).

Women of this age experience slowed metabolism (to their great frustrations) as well as lowered hormone production. For weight and mood, therefore, menopause and maturation are equal disasters. Your body will go completely "out of whack" compared to how it used to function. You'll likely put on weight despite the dietary choices you make, and you may feel there's no relief in sight. Don't be fooled, however! Things may have changed for you, but they won't be stagnant changes.

Essentially, women at the stage of menopause and beyond need to absorb less energy overall from their food, yet they need more protein to deal with the effects of aging. Vitamins B12 & D, calcium, and zinc will need to be boosted, while iron becomes less important for the aging female body. Vitamins C, E, A, & beta-carotene need to be increased too in order to fight off cancer, infection, disease, and more.

As the woman ages and matures even further, more things will change; mainly, she cannot bypass taking these important supplements any longer. In older and more mature women, the body's abilities to recognize hunger and thirst become muted, and dehydration poses a greater threat. Fewer calories are required for the older and more mature woman too, but she still needs to get as many nutrients as (if not more than!) the young woman does.

It seems that a younger woman can eat (relatively) what she wants and not worry about taking vitamins or supplements, but it is undeniable that the older woman will need this nutritional help to ensure longevity. Basically, health needs become more pressing for women at this age, as their bodies are less flexible and resistant to problems that may arise.

CHAPTER 12: SHOPPING LIST FOR YOU WHEN ON INTERMITTENT FASTING

Avocado is rich in omega-3s, which help your immune system and your body fight inflammation.

Beans & Lentils are great sources of protein and fiber, particularly for older women.

Blueberries are high in vitamin C and antioxidants that help protect the skin from pollutants, sun exposure, aging stress, and more.

Broccoli, Cauliflower, & Brussel Sprouts are all relatively high in lutein, which keeps your brain healthy and sharp!

Carrots are also rich in vitamin A as well as beta-carotene, which helps your vision later in life.

Cilantro might taste like soap to some, but it helps remove metals from your body that shouldn't be there. It's a great detoxifier for women of any age.

Cooked Tomatoes have a powerful antioxidant present that helps the skin heal from any kind of damage.

Dark Chocolate is packed with flavanols (which aid in the appearance of the skin and protect against the damage of the sun).

Edamame aids in bone health, cardiovascular healing, and eases into lowered estrogen levels with menopause.

Fortified Plant-Based Milk is a great non-dairy alternative to the "healing" animal milk you may know and love. They provide bone-supportive minerals and nutrients like calcium and vitamin D (as long as they're fortified!) without adding in the problematic nature of dairy to your healthy drink.

Ghee is a special form of clarified butter that is packed with healthy fats for skin health and detoxification.

Green Tea de-stresses the body and mind and blocks DNA from damage in many forms.

Manuka Honey is a special type of honey that's a powerful natural remedy for immune boost and skin health.

Mushrooms are high in vitamin D, which is so important for women of all ages.

Nuts are great at lowering cholesterol and fighting inflammation. They're also packed with fiber, protein, and micronutrients.

Oatmeal provides carbohydrates that encourage the release of serotonin, which keeps you feeling good.

Olives provide polyphenols and other essential phytonutrients that keep your DNA protected and your skin and body feeling and looking young.

Oranges, Lemons, & Limes, when juiced, provide the greatest source of healthy vitamin C you can imagine.

Papaya has many antioxidants, vitamins, and minerals that keep the skin elastic with fewer wrinkle lines.

Pineapples help maintain skin health, elasticity, and strength as you age.

Pomegranate Seeds are also high in antioxidants, and they're great at fighting free radical molecules that encourage the effects of aging on the body.

Red & Orange Bell Peppers have antioxidants and high vitamin C to help the skin retain its healthy shine while protecting it against pollutants and toxins.

Red Wine, when drunk in moderation, is a powerful tool to keep your heart healthy, lower cholesterol, and maintain muscle mass.

Saffron has anti-tumor, antioxidant, and other highly nutritious effects for the body.

Sesame Seeds will help you feel good through their high levels of calcium, magnesium, fiber, phosphorous, and iron.

Spinach & Other Leafy Greens work to protect the skin from sun damage while providing beta-carotene and lutein to solidify that effect.

Sweet Potato has more vitamin A than regular potatoes, which keeps your skin fresh and young-looking without lines and wrinkles.

Turmeric is great for the skin and for keeping the organs working in tip-top shape. The pigment curcumin also helps to heal DNA and prevent degenerative diseases.

Watercress is a happily hydrating green that's high in phosphorous, manganese, calcium, potassium, vitamins A, C, K, B1, and B2.

Watermelon works as a natural sun blocker when eaten and provides a great source of water to keep you hydrated.

Yogurt helps your cells stay young and is often probiotic, which is great for healthy gut flora and mood stabilization.

BEST FOODS & DIETS FOR PCOS

Whether or not you decide to attempt intermittent fasting with PCOS, however, please make sure to speak with your doctor first. And if you do decide to combine the two, make sure you seek the most healthful, nutrition-dense foods you can for breakfast. The biggest concern for women with PCOS trying IF is that they're simply worried about losing weight when their bodies are going through something much more complex than just weight gain. By ensuring your food choices are healthy and supportive, you will work to heal yourself as a whole rather than just one side-effect of PCOS. Some healthful foods that go well with the condition and side-effects of PCOS are as follows.

- Meats, Fish, & Eggs

- Cold Water Fish (esp. Salmon & Sardines)

- Healthy Fats

- Probiotics (both in drinks & foods)

- Non-Starchy Vegetables

- Fruit (with restriction – see below)

- Carbohydrates (with restriction)

- Whole Foods (generally)

- Natural, Unprocessed Foods

- High-Fiber Foods

- Leafy Greens

- Dark Red & Blue Fruits (esp. Blueberries, Blackberries, Cherries, & Red Grapes)

- Beans & Legumes

- Nuts

- Spices (esp. Turmeric & Cinnamon)

- Dark Chocolate (with restriction)

- Cruciferous Vegetables

- Squash (of all types)

- Anti-Inflammation Foods (i.e., Tomatoes, Kale, Spinach, Almonds, Walnuts, Olive Oil, Blueberries, Fatty Fish, Etc.)

- Green (& other flavors of) Tea

You may decide that intermittent fasting isn't right for you, given your condition, after all. In this case, you can still work to lose that pesky weight! You just might have to switch gears back to what's being eaten rather than when it's consumed. You'll want to make sure that you don't restrict too much from your diet, so (for example) a completely raw, plant-based diet might take too much from you when you still need a lot of what that diet could never provide. Be careful, too, about fad diets that you haven't researched into for yourself (such as the lectin-free and keto diets). Some diets that work well for people with PCOS are as follows.

Vegan Diet (or restricted-dairy Vegetarian Diet): If you're able to cut out meat in your diet (and interested in doing so), you might find that the Vegan Diet provides restriction of dairy in ways that help with your condition. However, you will need to avoid bingeing on gluten and soy substitutes as they are not friendly to people with PCOS. You could also try a Dairy-Restricted Vegetarian diet. There are certainly options to play around with until things feel right (or at least better) inside.

Dairy-Restricted Diet: A Dairy-Restricted Diet might be the best middle ground for someone in your shoes. You might not be interested in cutting meat out of your diet, but knowing that dairy is unhelpful, just focus on that. Cut out dairy completely or limit your intake to only once a day. The less you consume, the better, and it can happen one step at a time.

Gluten-Restricted Diet: Gluten adds to inflammation in the body, which makes things difficult for women with PCOS who already have a lot of inflammation in their bodies. What makes matters worse is that the more inflammation we have, the more insulin-resistant we become (bad!), and the more testosterone exists in our bodies (bad for you, PCOS lady!). The problem gets a little tougher because many gluten-free alternatives are super-refined, meaning that they're not good for your insulin levels either. So the trick will be to avoid or restrict gluten without going to gluten-free alternatives. That's going to be interesting...

No-GMO Diet: Highly modified food products like gluten and corn tend to aggravate conditions for women with PCOS, but another one that's less noticed is soy. Soy is hugely modified compared to its original existence as a seed and plant, but soy also makes hormonal issues for women with PCOS all the worse. Soy makes ovulation even more delayed for women, whether or not they have PCOS, so it really should be avoided along with other genetically-modified foods.

Sugar-Restricted Diet: Sugar, even in fruit, can be problematic for people with PCOS. Processed and refined sugar, in particular, is detrimental for women with PCOS who hope to get pregnant someday because they decrease the quality of their eggs, increase rates of miscarriage and reduce your sex drive as well. Even the fructose in fruits can make your insulin production wonky and contribute to weight gain if you overly rely on fruits in your diet. Try to cut out processed sugars but limit that fresh fruit consumption, too. Your situation will certainly be made better.

CHAPTER 13: MEALS PLAN FOR INTERMITTENT FASTING

Eating disorders are a real problem, and women are overwhelmingly more prone to developing them. So, how does all of this information relate to intermittent fasting, you may wonder? Well, my point is that the way intermittent fasting places emphasis on specific periods of fasting, followed by strict eating windows, it can sometimes cause women to develop an unhealthy obsession with food.

If your body is still getting used to going extended periods of time without eating, there is a greater likelihood that when the feeding window begins you will be so hungry that you overdo it. If you are really wanting to see results from following this protocol and are ashamed of yourself for consuming an excessive amount of food, the guilt you feel might even lead you to become bulimic, purging yourself to try and undo the situation. Likewise, if after adhering to intermittent fasting for some time and not seeing the results that you hoped for, you may start to feel like what you are doing is not enough. This can cause women to become more predisposed to developing anorexia.

When this happens, it is easy to see how someone may shorten their eating window far too much or barely eat any food at all during the allotted feeding time. Although women must be aware and cautious of these eating disorders when beginning intermittent fasting, this becomes even more important if they have any prior history of eating disorders, as the likelihood of relapsing increases substantially. To prevent any of these eating disorders from rearing their ugly head, one needs to make sure that their perspective is in the right place. The first thing you need to remember is that intermittent fasting is about becoming a healthier, happier version of you.

Remember all of the benefits you can enjoy that we discussed earlier? Well, these don't mean anything if you develop an extremely unhealthy relationship with food in the process. It is important that you keep in mind why you started it in the first place; to better yourself. The second thing to keep in mind is that you are a human being (shocker, right?). We are imperfect creatures with limited self-control; we make mistakes.

I can assure you that if you choose to begin intermittent fasting, there will be times that you make mistakes. Maybe that eating window just cannot wait, and you give in to the hot and ready sign at Krispy Kreme on your way home. Sometimes you may consume a few too many calories when those precious feeding hours begin. In nutrition, fitness, and even life in general, it is never the small, infrequent things that yield long term results. What you need to remember is that the things you do HABITUALLY are what will make or break you.

If you eat a terrible diet routinely and randomly decide to eat healthy for only one day, do you think you are going to immediately lose 10 pounds? Is going to the gym twice a year going to get you in fantastic shape and allow you to reach your fitness goals? Having said that, slipping up on your diet from time to time or missing a workout every once in a while is not going to ruin your weight-loss and exercise goals. Anything worth achieving, especially when it comes to your body, is not going to happen overnight.

However, if you consistently follow the intermittent fasting protocol or any other diet for that matter, then even with the minor setbacks that happen, you are still on the path to your goals! When it comes to intermittent fasting, you need to understand that this is merely a tool at your disposal that you are choosing to use to become a healthier person. You must never let something like this control you, after all, you are the one in control choosing to live this lifestyle, and you have the power to stop or change the rules at any time.

In your journey with intermittent fasting, it is of the utmost importance that you never lose sight of the big picture. Remember that food is not the most important thing in your life, and preoccupation with eating should never get in the way of the things that matter most to you. Although cruel, societal definitions and images portrayed by the media are giving us a horrible definition of what it means to be healthy. Most of the muscular men shown in movies and magazine covers are abusing harmful substances such as anabolic steroids, and a large number of women modeling the latest fashions are secretly suffering from the eating disorders that we discussed.

If you let it, comparing yourself to these people will do nothing but rob you of your joy and discourage you from trying to be your best. The only measuring stick that you should stand next to in your journey should be your former self. It is amazing how much fitness and nutrition mirror all of life itself. In everything you do, you should wake up every morning trying to improve yourself from the 'you' that fell asleep last night. Never let anyone tell you that you are not good enough and that you're not capable of reaching your health and wellness goals. You are more than capable of achieving them with the right amount of knowledge and commitment.

Intermittent fasting is a tried and true method of eating that human beings have been utilizing for thousands and thousands of years, without even really knowing the true extent of its benefits. When it comes to women's health and wellness, always remember that YOU are in control of your life. Modern media's definition of what you should look like and how you should eat is in your face everywhere you turn in your daily life. It is time to change the way that our society defines healthy eating and what it means to have an ideal physique. Do not let anyone or anything define who you are and what you can accomplish.

CHAPTER 14: SHARING INTERMITTENT FASTING WITH OTHERS

In our world today, the standard of beauty and what constitutes the ideal physique has promoted and even praised unrealistic expectations for men and women alike. Everywhere you look there are cover models on magazines with chiseled abs, models fitting perfectly in size zero dresses, actors in every movie with physiques the average person could probably never obtain. Being exposed to this sort of standard from every angle day after day can most definitely wear on our self-image and confidence.

As I said, this goes for both men and women, but I think we can all agree that women bear the brunt of this aspect of life. The media does its very best to make you believe that you cannot be considered pretty or in shape unless you mimic these unrealistic expectations presented to you in magazines and television. Sadly, this not only leads to lowered self-esteem in large numbers of women but sometimes it can escalate into health disorders.

To try and cope with these expectations, some individuals develop a severe eating disorder known as bulimia. This is a disorder where someone usually consumes a large amount of food, feels guilty, and then becomes so worried that it will be detrimental to their physique that they actually induce vomiting or take a large amount of laxatives, in a desperate attempt to reverse the situation. These methods are usually referred to as "purging." This disorder can wreak absolute havoc on the body. People with bulimia commonly have severe stomach distortion from overeating, electrolyte imbalance from severe dehydration, ulcers covering the lining of their esophagus from the constant stomach acid coming up from vomiting, and tooth decay also due to stomach acid. Although men and women both suffer from this disorder, women are much more prone to it. The United States Department of Health and Human Services reports that as many as 2% of women suffer from this eating disorder.

Another severe eating disorder many people suffer from is anorexia. This results in a person limiting their food intake to dangerously low levels for fear of gaining weight, exercising far too much in an attempt to burn calories. They often have a severely distorted body image in which they feel that they are obese when in reality they are far too thin. Once again, even though this disorder affects both men and women, it is predominately a female condition, with an estimated 1 in 20 women in the United States suffering from anorexia. This disorder also has terrible health implications such as heart problems, anemia, and extremely high-risk pregnancies.

CHAPTER 15: A BIT OF EXERCISE

When people picture themselves making better life choices, they often picture themselves eating better and then following this up with a lot of cardio and sit-ups. This, of course, can be a part of the ketogenic diet, but first, you need to change many of the ideas you probably have over exercise and dieting.

When the image of someone "dieting" springs to a person's mind, they often think of someone who is eating much less than average and following up this pitiful meal by working out for an hour. This model is not only unsustainable but ridiculous. We've already covered that the keto diet can be full of rich, enjoyable meals that will fuel your body and make you feel good. Exercise can be equally enriching.

Just in case you don't know, exercise is primarily fueled by glucose. When glucose is stored as glycogen, it is the glycogen stores that get burned when you do strenuous exercise. So, you may be wondering how exercising works on the keto diet, considering that you're switching your body over to burning fat.

Some people may read the fact that exercise burns glucose and think that exercise is impossible. Or that they shouldn't bother.

To be clear: you can get by without worrying about exercise. The majority of our health comes from what we eat, and as long as you're moving around a lot during the day in the form of walking and standing, you should be fine. Although exercise does have its health benefits. It helps make our bones stronger, enhances muscle growth and sustainability, and is good for the heart. So, implementing even just a light exercise routine is very beneficial.

There are four kinds of exercise you can do:

Aerobic: This is what is commonly known as cardio and is anything that's high intensity and lasts for over three minutes. It predominantly uses carbs as an energy source.

Anaerobic Exercise: this is what people consider interval training. It requires shorter bursts of energy, and carbs are once again its primary source of energy. Think of weight training or high cardio interval training.

Flexibility: this is anything that stretches your body. Think yoga or after workout stretches. This kind of exercise is great for your joints, improving your muscle range of motion, and helps prevent injuries.

Stability: think balancing exercises and core training. It improves alignment, strengthens muscles, and helps control movements.

What energy is burned really depends on the intensity of your workout, but the gist of it is this:

- Low-intensity: fat is used as energy

- High-intensity: glycogen is used as energy

Pretty simple, right?

However, that does mean that you need to consume more carbs if you do more high-intensity workouts. It goes back to the fact that the more you work out, the more carbs you need. You're going to have to adjust the carbs based on your lifestyle.

If you exercise more than three times a week, consider looking into a different kind of ketogenic diet, specifically the Targeted Keto Diet.

We already talked a bit about it before, but the idea is that you eat all your carbs around the time you work out. Eat 15 g to 30 g of carbs right before and right after. This gives your muscles glycogen to help your muscles recover, and any extra glucose will be burned away by the workout.

For the first few weeks of the keto diet, exercise will be pretty hard on your body. This means that for this time, you're going to have to take it easy, like with walks and light yoga. The longer your body gets used to burning fats for energy, the better you will feel. You will find your exercise performance will increase after a few weeks.

In the beginning, focus on the diet first, rather than the exercise. Feeding your body with the proper nutrients it needs and letting it adapt to the different fuel sources is more important, at first. After your body gets adjusted, you will find it much easier.

CONCLUSION

Throughout this book, we have discussed all of the ways in which you can start to include intermittent fasting in your life. As you can see, there are many health benefits besides just losing weight.

Many people, especially women, will want to lose weight throughout their lives because of the societal pressures put in place by capitalist industries. Once we become aware of this, it's easier to see the way that companies will feed off of our insecurities, trying desperately to get us to buy into things we don't need to lose weight in unhealthy ways.

Losing weight is important if you are overweight or obese, but it has nothing to do with your physical appearance. Reducing your weight will help reduce your risk for serious health conditions that come along with being out of shape, such as heart disease and even some cancers.

Apart from this, you want to extend your life and live it to the fullest, as it's the only one you'll ever have! You may as well do so in a healthy way that promotes autophagy and the consistent regeneration of new cells.

What is most important to remember moving forward is to listen to your body. You will have to push it sometimes, and there are days when you need to work through cravings. You'll be pushing yourself sometimes through these challenging thoughts, but never push yourself too far to where you feel like you're going to break!

If you have any health issues beyond just being out of shape, it's crucial you talk to your doctor. As we've discussed, fasting is safe, but for the average person. Other health conditions, such as diabetes, can be inflated by fasting. It doesn't mean that you will never be able to include this in your diet, but you might want to start with something else first.

Remember that fasting will help your body burn fat cells, but if you add too many fat cells again later on, then it will be hard to see the results that you want. If you want to lose weight and keep it off, it's time to work with your body.

Use the natural processes that are already inside of you. It's time to unlock these methods and remind yourself that you have everything that you need!

I have given you all that is needed to get started with this diet, and now it is time for you to take what you've learned and put it to good, practical use.

You deserve to have a happy and healthy body. If there is one thing that I want you to take away from this book, it is that your health is most important. Overall, you should feel good in your body, which will help your mind feel better, creating a perfectly content soul. Forget about looking good and just losing weight. Focus on feeling good! At the end of the day, what matters most is how you feel about yourself, and that can be done through healthy lifestyles that include intermittent fasting.

SIMPLY AUTOPHAGY

How to Leverage Your Body's Natural Intelligence to Reduce Inflammation, Slow Down Aging, Lose Weight Easily through Intermittent Fasting and Other Specific and Targeted Diets!

Josie Kidd

INTRODUCTION

Autophagy protects bone density and muscle mass. The mineral intake that you get after having autophagy can protect your bone density. The bones need certain minerals that are used to cure the excessive number of hurdles one gets while running. The minerals are given by autophagy, and you are able to get a stronger bone for life. If you are a bodybuilder and want to reap the benefits of the bone, then you have to accumulate more autophagy in you that can be very beneficial for you. The muscle mass can be secured in an acute manner if you tend to get more and more almonds and other alkaline dietaries. You have to be very lenient when you are having autophagy because the benefit of autophagy, such as muscle, muscle mass and bone density, will be instrumental for you. Just always look at the bright side of the diet, and you will feel very productive while you do it.

In today's world, tensions are like a haunting disease that wants to remain at your back for no reason. Everywhere you go, you get a tertiary level of tension. There is the tension of graduating, the tension of succeeding in life, the tension of getting a job, and the tension of whatnot. You believe that tension can be very successive for you, but in the latter, it turns out to be adverse. Scientists have claimed many medical drugs for their cure, but the only reasonable cure is the use of an alkaline diet. The enzymes that you get through vegetables lower the risk of your hyper blood tension, and then you can achieve all the relish of your lifestyle in no time. Also, your blood level starts to resonate with full capacity, and you will feel like a superman every place you go, therefore, hypertension and tense matters get an upper hand of resolution when you get to know the prospect of an alkaline diet.

Over time, our cells produce by-products and waste from the hard work that they are constantly doing. This microscopic bio-waste is collected in the cell, like an overflowing trash can. This happens when we eat too many sugars and carbohydrates, changing our insulin absorption and affecting our whole system's ability to function properly. When the cells are running slow because the waste is building up on account of a poor diet, lack of exercise, and our over-consumption of food daily, slowly over time, we begin to see the results: cancer, diabetes, inflammatory disease, cardiovascular disease, and rapid aging.

Our bodies are intelligent and know how to clean house and heal, especially if we create the right conditions for this process to occur. Autophagy is a self-healing mechanism at the cellular level that, when achieved, can change the health of your whole life.

CHAPTER 1: WHAT IS AUTOPHAGY?

This chapter will deal with the definition, the working of autophagy, the types of autophagy, and the usage of autophagy in the coming time. This chapter will also include the various formations of autophagy through which the people's way is moved forward in the direction. The contextualization of the book is as follows:

DEFINITION

According to Doctor Priya Khorana, the process of autophagy means the exit of food through the stomach, and it makes the metabolism look very clean. The cells that are used in this process are easily removed during this process, and later there is the rejuvenation of newer cells for healthy growth for humans. Auto means self, and the word phagy means eating. Therefore, autophagy means that the body will eat automatically, and with the passage of time, the old food will be removed.

By some authors, it is also related to self-devouring. This is the beneficial omen for your body and the process of self-devouring. The body cells are easily extinguished from the body thoroughly. The process of cellular repair also takes place in this context, and the overall body metabolism reaches its zeal. Thus, the use of cellular repair will make the body look better in the coming. The process of autophagy is a revolutionary self-preserving mechanism that helps in the elimination of carbon-related diseases in the human body.

For some, the definition is also contextualized as the process through which the cells of the body easily function in a better manner. There is also the removal of debris. It is referred to as the process of recycling and removing at the same time. The prolific medical scientist referred to it as the way of resetting your body, and the body aims to reach the better part of life. It is also a promotion of better toxin-related concepts of the body, and it will amplify the metabolism of the body in a perpetual manner.

WHY AUTOPHAGY WORKS

There is an ancient saying that the body will work if led with a proper mind. The use of autophagy helps to instill a proper mode of management for the people through which the persons are able to lead a happy life. The working of autophagy is also productive because it is able to give marvelous and potential results to the human body. It creates the possibility and creation of better cells that are quite great in their number, and they are able to curb strong measurements of disease prevention in them. There are many other benefits of it through which the body is able to receive better quality digestion and heat of hydration. There are numerous working mechanisms that are cultivated in the body through the use of autophagy. Since the use of autophagy brings about better changes in the human body, therefore, the use of autophagy works in the coming time, and it is much effective for the use of the human body.

AUTOPHAGY FOR HEALTH

There are five important ways through which autophagy works for the construction of health for the students and civilians. These ways help to restore the health factor for autophagy constructively.

1. EATING A HIGH FAT, LOW-CARB DIET

The eating of a high-fat triggers autophagy in the body. The use of high fat and its gestation ultimately exits some cells from the body through which the people are able to have a better understanding of the body in their dimension. The low carb diet will make you suit for autophagy as the process of elimination of cells will be random in the body, and the person will be able to give more value to its body. So, the intake of high fat will make the body have more leniency in it, and with the passage of time, the body will get rid of all the cells that make the body look pale and obstructive in the coming time.

2. GO ON A PROTEIN FAST

Autophagy will be helpful for the protein fast. Because in this fast you will be able to do a lot of mass exemption from the body. During the fast of the body, the people will be able to have a better comprehension of the body through which the protein of the body will go away, and the body will be given a better way of creating proteins in the coming time. Therefore, going on a protein fast will help to make the body a much better and more regulatory space.

3. PRACTICE INTERMITTENT FASTING

The concept of intermittent fasting is that the body has to take a lot of proteins from the human body, and there is a regular break from eating and drinking. There are time intervals through which the body is able to garner more food and water in the body. This time can be used to make the body look better and productive in the coming time. The use of strong fasting can make the body relax and have a sustainable work in the coming. So, if you want to attain a benefit from autophagy for health, then practice intermittent fasting.

4. EXERCISE REGULARLY

Exercising regularly can also initiate a fast rate of autophagy for you. Exercise helps to reduce fats allowing for more proteins to actually work in the body. The working of the body helps to maintain a strong pH value of the system, and the body is able to foment a healthier metabolism. This is a concept through which the autophagy of the body functions in a better way, and with the passage of time, autophagy tends to be sustainable in a better function.

5. DRINK A LOT OF WATER

Drinking a lot of water also helps you to maintain a stable metabolism of yourself through which you are able to have a yielding understanding of things around you. Drinking a lot of water makes the pH. value system aware of all the things happening around, and with the passage of time, the body is able to make healthier changes in the coming time. Drinking a lot of water will keep the diet clean and healthy, and it will make your body fit for any changes coming in the contemporary. Therefore, drinking a lot of water is crucial for you to maintain an autophagy state.

TYPES OF AUTOPHAGY

There are three types of autophagy. One is the macro-autophagy, micro-autophagy, and chaperone-mediated autophagy.

1. MACRO-AUTOPHAGY

Macro-autophagy is a type of autophagy in which the degradation of organelles occurs. It is a matured vesicle process. It is strongly recommended for the homeostasis process, in which the persons belonging to various paths and parallels are identified in the human being for a perpetual state of mind. The use of macro-autophagy can be illustrated in many ways of the world. The uses are very much in use these days. The use of microautophagy can be related to many uses like the cure of brain diseases and brain coverages. The use of macroautophagy has many abilities embedded in it. It can be used to treat neurodegenerative diseases in people. The disease-linked aggresomes can be used in many uses to make the fossils and the human platelets working in a better way. Macroautophagy can also be constructed in many ways possible for the people coming forward. Therefore, Macroautophagy is the branch of autophagy, which deals with the process of clearing the established fats in the body.

2. MICRO-AUTOPHAGY

The construct of microautophagy is different from two types of autophagy, which are macro and chaperone-mediated autophagy. These autophagias help the micro people and the lysosomal action to be easily overridden by the people and the body state. This practice is adopted by many people abroad, and it can also be found with many people and other doctors to be precisely relevant. This practice is very important for the functioning of cells, and it helps to give more emphasis to the extermination of diseases in the coming time. Cytoplasmic material is trapped in the cells of the people, and the people are able to manifest the uses of autophagy properly. This process is also used for nitrogen deprivation, and it can lead to strong illustrations of people effectively. There are three special cases of a selective microautophagic pathway: micropexophagy, piecemeal microautophagy of the nucleus, and micromitophagy. These phages make the body of the human being emerged from the ashes.

There are very important functions of micro-autophagy. There are used for nutrient recycling. This is done for the degradation of lipids. It regulates the composition of the vacuolar membrane. There are many mechanisms of glycogen in it. The pathway that comes through micro-autophagy helps to create a link with the multivesicular bodies, endocytic, membrane proteins, and the use of strong organelle size. There is also non-selective micro-autophagy in this regard. There is membrane invagination, vesicle formation, vesicle expansion, vesicle degradation, and selective micro-autophagy. These invaginations help to create a better formation of body cells for the persons coming forward, and with the passage of time, the body is able to eat all the fats and vitamins of the structure effectively. This practice is of strong use and pertinence and can be regarded effectively in the coming time.

The process of selective micro-autophagy can be observed in all types of eukaryotic cells. On the other hand, this is also commonly observed in yeast cells. Therefore, micro-autophagy helps to create a cluster of better engines for the coming community.

3. CHAPERONE-MEDIATED AUTOPHAGY

This chaperone-mediated autophagy helps to give more ideas to the process of autophagy. This is referring to the selection of chaperone dependent selection. The selection of soluble proteins is taken into account. The cytosolic proteins are targeted to lysosomes and are directly related to the concept of lysosome membrane without the requirement of the formation of additional values. The proteins that want to make the structure of CMA are cytosolic proteins and proteins from other compartments. There are some compartments that discuss the nature of CMA, and they are worthy of being discussed here. These are the compartments that tend to make the working of the cells more functional and linear in their working. There is selectivity of proteins, and the proteins are able to make the manufacture of the engine more compatible. The CMA can be of many uses and regards of the people, and the people are able to blend with the work coherently.

The proteins that participate in the CMA are more likely to be engulfed by the main cell of the body. First, there is the degradation of cells, there is the presence of cytosolic protein in the making, there is the formation of amino acid in work, there is lysosome-associated work of the protein type A in the formation, there is a receptor for the membrane of the formation of the work, the two isoforms are found in the cells of the body through which one has to trade genes to the people coming ahead, there are substrates that deal with the process of working for the people and then there are translocation purposes that make the deal of CMA more workable. There is an artificial use of people that do not cater properly to the formation of the work, and with the passage of time, there is a better comprehension thing coming forward.

The matter comes to the people of the formation in a close manner, and this thing helps to bind the CMA more effectively for the people. Therefore, the use of a close manner can be sorted out more periodically in the coming time. There are some limitations to the CMA process. One is the binding of the substrate of the people coming forward, and with the passage of time, the CMA tends to be more linear with time. There are some levels of constraints to the process of CMA as well. With the passage of time, the CMA tends to devolve, and if one wants to maintain a proper outlook of CMA, then there need to be some limitations. The levels of CMA are easily utilized, and they are made under some uncertainties for the people. The people in these uncertainties are not able to proceed with CMA, and hence, they are able to come stringently ahead.

These are three types of autophagias discussed above in an effective manner.

Once you are able to identify the process by understanding the different ways autophagy can occur inside the cell, you can picture the process and connect the dots with why you might want to activate autophagy in your body. If you have never fasted, experienced ketosis through your food intake, or had any kind of exercise routine, then you are likely walking around with some very cluttered cells that need some serious cleanup. Autophagy is always happening on some level; however, when you are not creating circumstances to help it occur optimally, then it is only working at a moderate to low level of efficiency. There are many ways that initiating autophagy can improve your health and prevent serious or chronic health conditions later in life.

Even though self-degradation occurs in nearly every organism's cells as a survival mechanism, from yeast to humans, there are three different ways in which the cell delivers what it longer needs to the degradation vesicle – the lysosome. These can be distinguished depending on how the cell forms the lysosome, the number of steps required, and the cargo contained in the vesicles.

Most of the cellular waste is eliminated through macroautophagy, which has long been considered the default pathway and by far the most studied. During macroautophagy, cells use their own membranes to form two types of vesicles: one called autophagosome, which captures any product and the lysosome, containing enzymes that help speed up the recycling process. Microautophagy is a more straight-forward way to achieve the same result, however, it's not molecule-specific: any substance can be removed from the cell's interior and directly delivered to the lysosome. Recently, studies described a subtype of microautophagy that helps the cell integrate proteins produced at the endoplasmic reticulum, proving that autophagy is not an exclusively catabolic mechanism.

On the opposite end of the spectrum, we have chaperone-mediated autophagy, which only targets protein into the lysosome. Each protein is assigned to a signaling molecule that is then recognized by chaperones included in the degradation of the vesicle membranes. In some cases, chaperones can also recognize transcription factors, proteasomes, and proteins involved in cellular transportation systems. For this to happen, proteins must present a very specific structural pattern, the KFERQ motif. Without this motif, chaperone-mediated autophagy cannot progress normally, as it's essential for the uptake and unfolding process that occurs at the lysosome.

CHAPTER 2: WAYS TO INITIATE AUTOPHAGY

You may be on board with the idea of having your cells eat each other, but are probably now wondering how you would go about doing it. Or more accurately, how you would trigger your body to kick start this process for you. The good news is that autophagy is a response to stress. This means that when you stress your body in certain ways, the process is triggered. But not all stress will do the trick. When you add a little bit of extra stress to your body, the self-consumption process is elevated. This added stress can be uncomfortable at the moment, but the idea is that this little bit of extra stress can lead to incredible, long-term joy. Adding more stress in a controlled manner can result in amazing benefits to your body. There are three primary ways to induce your autophagy process; exercise, fasting, and decrease your carbohydrate intake significantly.

EXERCISE

You have probably heard for a long time now that diet and exercise are the keys to a long and healthy life. This is no different, and the science to back up this is here for you in the first and second chapters. Exercise stresses your body at the moment. This is why people have pains after a hard workout, grunt when it is challenging, and sweat. When your muscles work hard, they get little tears in them that need to be repaired. Your body responds to these tears quickly, and while repairing the damage you just did, the body makes the muscle stronger so it can resist any future "damage" you might inflict upon it. You may not think of exercising as a way to clean out your cellular buildup of toxins, but it's one of the most common and popular ways to renew your cells. This helps explain why you feel so fresh and rejuvenated after a good, hard workout.

In one study on mice with highlighted autophagosomes, the researchers found that after they ran on a treadmill for 30 minutes their autophagy process was dramatically increased. An autophagosome is a resulting structure in the autophagy process. It forms around the damaged or toxic part of the cell and removes it to be disposed of, leaving behind the healthy parts of the cell. The increase in exercise provided evidence that these became more efficient and frequent than when the mice for less active. And it did not just increase the rate of autophagy while exercising! The increased rate of self-consumption continued for 80 minutes after stopping exercising. While there are no concrete studies or information regarding how much or how often a human should exercise to increase autophagy, it is clear the relationship exists in humans as well. Dr. Daniel Klionsky, a University of Michigan cellular biologist, explains that it is hard to determine the level of exercise a human must undergo to trigger their autophagy process, but there are so many clear benefits to exercise that no matter what you do, it will help support your body on some level. The best assumption to make in this case is to engage in more intense exercise regimens a few times a week for the best results. This is for general health benefits, but will also be the best amount of controlled stress on your body to trigger your autophagy.

FASTING

Cleanses that introduce any form of food or drink besides water into the body will actually prevent the trigger of autophagy, not allowing the body to effectively cleanse itself of toxins, as desired on a cleanse.

Instead, simply skipping a meal or two or three can be the best stress on the body that triggers autophagy, offering a true cleanse. Your body will probably not like it at the moment, but the benefits will be something it will enjoy for a long time. Research has shown, over and over again, that engaging in an occasional fast can help you lower risks of various illnesses like heart disease and diabetes. The reason for these benefits that medical professionals and scientists claim is because of autophagy.

There are several studies that have been published that specifically look at fasting, autophagy, and brain health. It is clear there is a distinct connection between lowering the risk of developing a neurodegenerative disease, like Parkinson's disease or Alzheimer's disease, when you engage in short-term fasts. Other studies reveal that intermittent fasts help support proper brain function, brain structure, and neuroplasticity. This is what helps your brain learn new information easier. While this information is exciting, it is not completely clear if autophagy is the reason, and most of these studies are conducted on animals. While the benefits are promising, they are not always applicable to human subjects.

There are a variety of adaptations for intermittent fasting, and it is something that can fit into almost anyone's life because of this. You can choose to abstain from eating food anywhere between 12 to 36 hours in a stretch, always drinking a lot of water during the fast. You can also engage in moderate to light physical activity during this time to help your body upregulate the results, but it is not typically advisable to engage in intense workouts during a fasting period. In addition, you can choose to fast only during certain times of the year, a certain day of the month, or one or more days a week.

DECREASE YOUR INTAKE OF CARBOHYDRATES

Fasting on a regular basis can be a challenge for many people, especially if you are used to constantly eating. In addition, this is contradictory to a lot of popular advice available now, encouraging people to eat little meals consistently throughout the day to boost metabolism. What research has shown, however, is that eating constantly does not keep your metabolism and hunger "satisfied" but rather creates a constant "hunger" hormone that keeps you wanting to eat and eat. Instead, when you fast, you learn the difference between true hunger and a triggered response at the time you normally eat a meal. You break your body of these habits and encourage it to focus on your cellular repair and fat-fuel burning instead. If you are having trouble getting into an intermittent fasting schedule, you can mimic the benefits in another way by decreasing your intake of carbohydrates.

This similar process is called ketosis. A lot of people who work out regularly or are looking to improve their long-term health and well-being have been turning to this type of eating regimen. The concept aims to significantly reduce the carbs that are consumed, so your body must use the fat for fuel instead of injected glucose from the conversion of the carbs. When your body enters into ketosis, it mirrors a lot of the same changes to your metabolism that autophagy offers. You get to enjoy the benefits of fasting without having to complete fast. In addition to the similar benefits to your metabolism, ketosis has been shown to help you maintain healthy body weight, protect your muscle mass, prevent and fight tumors, lower your risk of type-2 diabetes, minimize the risk of neurological diseases, and treat some brain disorders, like epilepsy. For example, in one recent study, more than 50% of the children with epilepsy that followed this diet experienced more than half the frequency of seizures than their peers not following the diet.

In addition to removing a lot of the carbs, you increase your intake of healthy fat. Most of your calories, up to 70%, come from fat on the Keto diet. This means eating a lot of meat, avocado, peanut butter, to name a few. Protein is up to 30% of your daily caloric intake. If you have room for carbs, you need to keep them to less than 50 grams every day. This is an extreme diet that many people get used to over time. If you can, being with a mix of fat/protein/carbs with your carb intake not exceeding 30% of your daily caloric intake and work back from there. Some find this regimen of eating more challenging than fasting, so it is wise to look into and try out what method works best for you in triggering your autophagy response.

If you are still looking at these three primary methods for triggering autophagy and wondering if there are other, easier ways, you will be discouraged to find that there are none. There will be a lot of money when researchers find a way to trigger autophagy or mimic it in a synthetic form like a pill, and it is being researched and considered now, but this is a long way off. Until the process is better understood, it is not possible to chemically induce the process in a human body. It is also unwise to turn to synthetic and chemical methods to avoid dieting and exercise for your well-being. It is also important to note that there are anti-epilepsy drugs being developed to mirror the state of ketosis in the body. If those become available, it is probable that people will begin taking them to mimic autophagy in the body instead of approaching it through traditional diet and exercise methods.

Keep in mind that the process of ketosis in the body is complex, as the process of autophagy. The idea that a single pill can mimic this entire, intricate, and complex process is unrealistic. The stress required to enter ketosis, for example, may be an integral part of the process. This means you will need to still exert effort and energy to get the pill to work in any form. It is also likely that the pill will only encourage one or two of the benefits of ketosis for a person suffering from epilepsy and not target any other benefits of ketosis. Yes, the three methods of activating autophagy and ketosis listed above all require effort, and it is important to also remember that you do not need to do each of them every day to get the results and benefits. Just a couple of hours a week or month can do the trick for supporting your cellular health.

Finally, there is a lot of published research available to show the indication of the various benefits of autophagy as well as how to activate it in a healthy way. The little bit of short-term and controlled stress can lead to controlled and systematic self-destruction so you can end up living a longer, healthier life. It is an ancient survival process that is designed to help the body in times of stress, like when your ancestors had to go days between meals that they hunted to feed themselves and their family. Starvation and physical exertion have the ability to kill you, but over millions of years, human bodies have evolved to turn those "bad" situations into something that can actually help you.

The molecular nature of autophagy was first discovered in budding yeast Saccharomyces cerevisiae as a model structure, functioning in all eukaryotic organisms but not in prokaryotes. Autophagic activity is necessary for the improvement of cellular homeostasis and energy balance.

A lot of evidence relates to malfunctions in autophagic processes to most clinically applicable diseases, including neurodegeneration, autoimmunity, cardiovascular disease, and diabetes. The creation of autophagy-focused therapies will rely on an extensive understanding of the benefits, and possible results, of changing autophagic activity.

Different forms of autophagy have been differentiated using the cargo is degraded. The most extensively researched type of autophagy –macro-autophagy reduces huge sizes of the cytoplasm and cellular organelles. Also, the selection of individual substrate classes, cytoplasmic organelles, protein aggregates, and bacteria requires special adaptors that identify the cargo and focuses on the autophagosome membrane. Other types of autophagy comprise macroautophagy, which requires the direct surrounding of cytoplasmic material through inward folding of the lysosomal membrane, and chaperone-mediated autophagy (CMA).

While autophagy is a degradative channel, it also takes part in biosynthetic and secretory processes. Since autophagy plays a big role in most essential cellular functions. It is not a surprise that autophagic dysfunction is related to multiple forms of human diseases.

Misfolded proteins have a tendency to create insoluble compounds that are dangerous to the cells. To solve this problem, the cells rely on autophagy.

Why autophagy is special, the response depends on the degree of flexibility of autophagosome size and selection of cargo. Autophagy can support degradation en masse for numerous and different forms of substrates allowing cells to quickly and effectively build up recycled basic building materials in the face of a broad type of nutritional deficiencies. Besides this, autophagy is the only medium that is capable of degrading whole organelles, randomly or in a targeted style. This is a critical procedure for regulating homeostasis in the complex landscape of the eukaryotic cell. This process authenticates a quality control mechanism that is important for counteracting the negative effects of aging. Autophagy refers to a dynamic, multi-step process that consists of autophagosomes development, depletion of the autophagic substrate, and autolysosome development. The development of autophagosomes, a thin membrane vesicle that surrounds cytosolic components into lysosomes for depletion and recycling, represents autophagy. During the time of autophagy stimulation, the cytoplasmic type of microtubule-related protein 1 light chain LC3 is lapidated and admitted to the autophagosomes. LC3 II, which is the lapidated type of LC3, is connected to the autophagosome membrane, which makes LC3 conversion a must for autophagosome development. The popularly used assay for tracking autophagic flux is the turnover of LCB, which measures the content using autophagic flux. But this method is time-consuming and labor-intensive, and the results are usually in different experimental settings and difficult to interpret. Understanding the need for a strong method to highlight autophagic compartments with little straining of endosomes and lysosomes is a critical approach for tracking autophagy and approximating the autophagic flux in active cells.

Now, let us examine the important benefits of autophagy in detail.

Although "self-eating" may look like a bad idea, it can be a source of youth and for your cells to regenerate. The phrase "autophagy" is a state for our cells to switch to repair damage and heal. This healing state is stimulated when we need to fight infection, save energy, and repair damage. Read on to discover why autophagy matters in your life.

AUTOPHAGY DECREASES THE RATE OF NEURODEGENERATIVE DISEASES

A lot of brain aging diseases take a lot of time to develop because they are the outcome of proteins in and around your brain cells that don't work right. Autophagy assists cells in cleaning up the proteins that don't do their work, and they are less likely to add. For example, autophagy removes amyloid in Alzheimer's disease and α-synuclein in Parkinson's disease. There is an explanation why dementia is believed to be at par with diabetes: the constant high blood sugar controls autophagy from activating, making it difficult to prevent these cells from clutter.

AUTOPHAGY CONTROLS INFLAMMATION

Autophagy stimulates a "Goldilocks" degree of inflammation by quelling the immune response you require. Autophagy can boost inflammation when an invader is available by stimulating the immune system to attack. In most cases, autophagy reduces inflammation from your immune response by halting the signals that trigger it.

AUTOPHAGY BOOSTS THE PERFORMANCE OF MUSCLES

As you build microtears and inflame muscles while exercising, the muscles need repair. The demand for energy increases. Your muscle cells will respond to this by getting into autophagy to decrease the energy needed to use the muscle and enhance the balance of energy to lower the risk of future damage.

AUTOPHAGY MAY ENHANCE THE QUALITY OF LIFE

The advantages of anti-aging may appear to be too good to be true, but the truth is more than the outer layer of the skin. Since the 1950s, scientists have been researching the process of autophagy, but recent studies have disclosed more about how it enhances cellular health. Rather than consuming new nutrients, the cells undergo autophagy to recycle the damaged parts they have, eliminate toxic material and fix themselves up. When your cells repair on their own, they work better, and they can work like younger cells. You may have noticed that some people have a very separate chronological and biological age. The degree of damage a body has taken and how it has managed to repair plays a big role in these differences.

AUTOPHAGY BOOSTS THE HEALTH OF THE SKIN

The cells that you expose to the world experience a lot of damage from air pollution, cold, chemicals, heat, humidity changes, and physical damage. That is the reason why it doesn't appear worse for wear. Once the cells of your skin hold toxins and damage, they start to age in place. Although your body creates new cells, autophagy can assist repair the current ones so that you glow well. Skin cells fight bacteria that may destroy the body, so it is important to support them as they clean the clutter.

AUTOPHAGY ENHANCES YOUR DIGESTIVE HEALTH

The cells inside your gastrointestinal tract are always triggered to function. In fact, a large percentage of your feces are your cells. With the help of autophagy, your digestive cells can repair and restore, clean themselves of junk, and activate the immune system as required. Since a chronic immune system within the gut can exhaust and inflame your bowels, an opportunity to repair, rest and recover is crucial to your health. Stimulate autophagy using a schedule that supports an extended overnight fast, and you can offer your gut space it requires to heal.

FIGHT INFECTIOUS DISEASE

Autophagy can help accept an immune response when required. Next, the process of autophagy can eliminate specific microbes directly from the inside cells like Mycobacterium tuberculosis, or even viruses like HIV. Autophagy can still eliminate the toxins generated by infections, which is necessary for foodborne illness.

AUTOPHAGY CAN BOOST A HEALTHY WEIGHT

Below are unique benefits of autophagy that create a healthy body:

- Autophagy demands fat-burning to be turned on but spares protein. On a very long fast, you will lose a protein mass, but in short fasting periods, you can stimulate autophagy, spare protein, burn fat, and receive all the benefits of a leaner and fitter you.

- Autophagy suppresses unnecessary inflammation. Chronic inflammation increases insulin, resulting in more weight storage and less inflammation that assist in decreasing the percentage of insulin.

- Autophagy decreases toxins inside the cell body. As long as you can remove toxins, they are less likely to require fat cells to store them.

- Autophagy permits metabolic efficiency by repairing the sections of cells that make and package proteins and synthesize energy, which is important when cells require to shift to fat-burning for energy.

IT REDUCES THE DEATH OF CELLS

Compared to cell death, the death of a cell is messy and builds garbage to clean up. Your body awakens inflammation to perform the clean –up. The higher the percentage of cells that repair themselves before they are damaged beyond repair, the less effort your body put into cleaning old cells and regenerating new ones. Minimal inflation is involved in regenerating tissues. You can make use of this energy to substitute cells that require continuous renewal, such as digestive cells. Although there are specific cells that need to be turned over a lot, not all cells need this. A lot of repair with minimal cleanup is a huge mix of success. While there are a lot of health benefits you can gain, it is a repair response to stress.

As we close on this chapter, autophagy performs two main roles. First, it removes damaging materials and foreign invaders. Secondly, it synthesizes cellular materials for energy during times of starvation. Improper control of autophagy is a big factor for numerous diseases like diabetes, autoimmune diseases, cancer, and infections. Not only does it eliminate damaged materials-it also activates senescence and enhances the cell present antigens on its surface. Researchers have started to establish autophagy as a critical process in both pathology and physiology.

CHAPTER 3: ANTI-INFLAMMATORY DIET BASICS

There are many forms of inflammation in the body. Some can be temporary, some chronic. Some forms that start as temporary may turn into a chronic condition. Along with multiple forms of inflammatory conditions, there are also as many opinions or more on how to treat them, bring down discomfort levels, or even just generally work to make you feel better.

So how do you pick and choose as to what is the best way for you to address whatever inflammatory condition you or a loved one may be experiencing? As with any medical condition, the first thing to do is to discuss it with your doctor. Even for those who prefer not to follow a more allopathic route (via western M.D., etc. solutions), let's face it—at the very least, our medical practitioners have worked and studied very hard at finding the various ways to make us feel better. Dr. Google is not always going to have the best answers for us or may have too many conflicting and confusing answers, leaving us lost to wade through a myriad of information mingled with misinformation.

What does this mean for those who want to be proactive in their health and supplement other treatments with additional avenues to help make themselves feel better? It means that you need to learn more about the health condition with which you are facing, how it affects you on different levels, and what additional options might be available to you.

Luckily, there are many aspects of anti-inflammatory conditions that can be addressed in a beneficial manner with a few simple lifestyle changes.

This is not to say that these are cures, but rather, they can be beneficial toward pain reduction and ease of living. In the case of this guide, the discussion will be focused on not only the dietary aspects of the equation but also as a well-rounded aspect from which you can attack your chronic issues from all sides. Diet can be looked at as more than just the food you put into your body. It is the nourishment provided to the body, something you experience repeatedly. Repetition creates habits. When dealing with chronic inflammation, it is necessary to break old, bad habits that increase the inflammation and replace them with a habitual diet of new and good habits that help you to feel better!

While there are some very basic steps that will help many or even most people, the first understanding you need in order to create fewer frustrations in any pursuit of lifestyle changes is that not everything will work for everyone. You could even be one of those people for whom nothing seems to work. It can happen. The closer look that you take at how your body actually *does* work in conjunction with the diagnosis for the condition you are facing, the more readily you stand the chance of finding what *does* work for you.

Sometimes the search for relief means a series of trials and errors. It is how research is done. Regardless of how frustrating this can be, it can help to take a positive outlook. You may not always find the answer you seek, but what you may find is what doesn't work for you. It is a process of elimination that can help in your search for a better quality of life. So don't get discouraged. Consider every step as a step in a positive direction. Learning what doesn't work for you can be just as important as what does. It will help you tailor your solutions specifically to you and your health and well-being.

As human beings with a myriad of genetic make-ups, backgrounds, areas, and conditions under which we have been raised or currently live, additional and/or multiple medical conditions, along with so many other influencing factors, we are each unique. How could it be any different in what will and will not work to make you feel better?

The pages to follow within this guide are designed to help you better understand how inflammatory conditions affect your overall body and health, why things generally do and do not work to make you feel better, and overall, to help you better understand your own body so, in turn, you can find what helps to make your body *feel* better.

As you step through the basics on the pages within this guide, take the time to learn about yourself. No one source is going to be the definitive "go-to" for everyone, but hopefully, you will find something to take away and make your journey on your way back to feel a better more positive and pleasant experience.

MOST BENEFICIAL FOODS AND BEST ANTI-INFLAMMATORY SUPPLEMENTS

Many conditions can be traced back to inflammation. Joint pain, autoimmune disorders, irritable bowel syndrome (IBS), mood imbalances, acne, and eczema are just a few conditions that can be linked back to inflammation. Once the origin of inflammation is identified, an anti-inflammatory diet can help ease symptoms, and certain foods and supplements can help lessen the inflammation in your body. In this chapter, we'll list some of the best minerals and beneficial antioxidants found in foods and supplements to add to your arsenal to fight inflammation. This list is arranged in alphabetical order to make it easier to use as a reference tool.

BLUEBERRIES

Blueberries make the list as an antioxidant superfood. This dark, delicious fruit may be small, but it's crammed with antioxidants and phytoflavinoids. These tiny berries are high in potassium and vitamin C and work as an anti-inflammatory to aid in lowering the risk of heart disease and cancer. Strawberries, raspberries, and blackberries also contain anthocyanins, which provide anti-inflammatory effects.

AVOCADO

Avocados are packed with potassium, magnesium, and fiber. This savory fruit is another superfood rich in antioxidants and anti-inflammatory properties. They provide a great source of healthy unsaturated fat and are packed with potassium, magnesium, and fiber.

COENZYME Q10

Coenzyme Q10, also known as CoQ10, is another antioxidant that has been shown to have anti-inflammatory properties. It is found naturally in avocados, olive oil, parsley, peanuts, beef liver, salmon, sardines, mackerel, spinach, and walnuts.

GINGER

Ginger is comparative to the fact that it contains powerful anti-inflammatory compounds known as gingerols. Ginger root is found in the produce section at your grocery store and is available as a potent antioxidant supplement that helps prevent the oxidation of a damaging free radical called peroxynitrite. Ginger adds flavor to your favorite stir-fry, can be made into ginger tea, or can be taken as a supplement.

GLUTATHIONE

Glutathione is another antioxidant that fights free-radicals with anti-inflammatory properties. This is available as a supplement and is also available naturally in plant foods, including apples, asparagus, avocados, garlic, grapefruit, spinach, tomatoes and milk thistle.

MAGNESIUM

Magnesium is a mineral supplement that can help reduce inflammation for those with low magnesium, which is linked to stress. Statistics suggest an estimated 70% of Americans are deficient in this mineral, which is surprising since it is readily available in a number of foods, including dark leafy greens, almonds, avocado, and many legumes.

SALMON

Salmon is rich in anti-inflammatory omega-3s. It is better to eat wild-caught than farmed. It is best to try to include oily fish in your diet two times a week, and if you're not a fan of fish, then try a high-quality fish oil supplement.

VITAMIN B

People with low levels of vitamin B6 have a tendency to have high levels of C-reactive protein, which, as was mentioned in chapter 2, is a measure of inflammation in the body. B vitamins, including B6, can be found in vegetables like broccoli, bell peppers, cauliflower, kale, and mushrooms. It is also available in meats, including chicken, cod, turkey, and tuna.

Folate (B-9 in natural form) and folic acid (a synthetic form of B-9) is another B vitamin linked to the reduction of inflammation. A brief Italian study submits that even daily, short-term low dosages of folic acid supplements can lessen inflammation in overweight people. Folate is found in foods like asparagus, black-eyed peas, dark leafy greens, and lima beans.

VITAMIN D

Estimates suggest two-thirds of the people living in the U.S. are deficient in vitamin D. It's another vitamin that helps reduce inflammation, and getting insufficient amounts is linked to a range of inflammatory conditions. This vitamin is unique in that we get it naturally when we spend time in the sunshine with the important spectrum is ultraviolet B (UVB). It is also available as a supplement and is available in foods like egg yolks, fish, and organ meats, as well as foods that are supplemented with it. When choosing a Vitamin D supplement, look for Vitamin D3, which is the most bioavailable form of the vitamin. The ideal amount for supplementation is 5000IU per day, and many of these pills cost less than $7 for a 3 month supply.

VITAMIN E

Another potent antioxidant, this vitamin can aid in lessening inflammation. It is available as a quality supplement or can be found naturally in nuts and seeds and vegetables like avocado and spinach.

VITAMIN K

There are two kinds of vitamin K: K1 and K2. K1 is found in leafy greens, cabbage, and cauliflower. K2 is available in eggs and liver. This vitamin helps reduce inflammatory markers and may help to fight osteoporosis and heart disease.

CHAPTER 4: FOODS THAT REDUCE METABOLIC INFLAMMATION

Becoming healthier and fitter should be a primary goal that anyone should follow. Autophagy can help you achieve this goal, as it's responsible for destroying and recycling old and damaged cell parts, in order for your body to work better. It is usually linked with the fat burning process, as autophagy happens when the body runs on fat. It basically actions on the fat cells, in order to get the energy required for your brain and body. Ketosis and fasting can be intertwined, as ketosis is regarded as the first phase of Intermittent Fasting, during which ketones levels are higher. Ketosis is not the same thing as the keto-adaption process.

The first term describes a metabolic state with appropriate levels of ketones and blood sugar. During this phase, the insulin level and blood sugar decreases, whilst the ketones levels are increasing. This is generated by glucose deprivation, meaning that it took quite a while since the body last had its glucose required for energy. This substance can be found in all the carbs (and proteins as well) and is the primary source of energy for the body under "normal circumstances."

Speaking of glucose intake, the modern-day diet relies heavily on carbs because we mainly consume processed food. This means that the body mainly uses the glucose from the carbs, but the big problem is that it simply can't burn all the glycogen it gets, mainly because of the high carb intake, but also because of the passive lifestyle. Nowadays, around

70% of the diseases known to humans are caused by the food we eat, and high amounts of carbs can be blamed for this situation. In urban communities, where most people live, it's a little difficult to find natural and organic food, as everywhere you are bombarded by processed food. The sad truth is that most of the food we eat today is processed, and this comes with very high levels of carbs. What's even worse is that these types of food have little to nothing nutritional value and cause addiction. In order to cover your daily nutritional needs, you have to eat more, but this means a caloric boom.

Processed food is more caloric dense than nutrient-dense, and this is a major disadvantage. When people are facing increased risks of chronic diseases like type 2 diabetes, heart, stomach, liver, and kidney diseases, it's clear that something has to be done to change the way we eat and also what we eat. Studies indicate that in order to become healthier and also thinner, you would need to decrease the glucose level when eating. This can happen by cutting down on carbs and, in some cases, also means protein limiting. When not burned, glucose gets stored in your blood, increasing the insulin and blood sugar level. Carbs consumption is like a vicious circle, as you easily get hungry after consuming food rich in carbs, and you are craving for more. But these meals come with strings attached, as you will get higher glucose levels and eventually higher blood sugar and insulin level. In order to make a radical change, you will need to make your body burn fat, not glucose. As you probably already have blood sugar, you will need to stop eating so many carbs, and therefore you will have less glucose to worry about. You can achieve this through fasting (restraining yourself from food) or through a special diet.

Traditional fasting means not consuming any food at all; some would not consume anything at all, just like religious fanatics during a special period, the Ramadan in the Islamic religion can be a perfect example. By not consuming anything at all, you are allowing your body to use the available glucose to be burnt, and once it has burned it all, the body will have to switch the energy source from glucose to fat. As the glucose level is decreasing, the same happens with the insulin level, setting it free to do its job and regulate the blood sugar.

The body easily adapts to such changes, and since its glucose reserves are running out, it has to figure out a way to use a different fuel type. That's where ketones step in, which is the necessary tool to break down fat cells and release the energy from them. You need to easily make the difference between ketosis and the keto-adapted process, as ketosis represents the metabolic state during which the ketone bodies are multiplying. The keto-adapted process is responsible for switching the energy source from glucose to fat. You can be in a ketosis state but still not running on fats and ketones for fuel.

Intermittent Fasting is more of a self-discipline process because it's about planning when to eat than what to eat. Limiting the feeding window to a limited amount of hours can give time for the body to process the food and use it for energy. However, when the body has already processed the food it has consumed, and it's not receiving anything else, it will start to look for a different alternative as fuel. The fat tissue is the most "to hand" option, and ketones can help extract the energy from it. If daily fasting has feeding and a fasting window, these terms are not the same with the fed and fasted state. The fed state represents the period of time required by your body to process the food it consumed, whilst the fasted state refers to the period after the fed state, during which the body doesn't have to process any food, and it's also not receiving any nutrients at all.

The fasted state starts approximately 12 hours after the last meal, and, coincidence or not, that's when ketosis starts. In the fasted state, the ketones levels are increasing rapidly, whilst the blood sugar and insulin levels are decreasing. At this point, the body doesn't have available glucose to burn, and it's looking for alternative fuel. Also, this is the right moment to apply stress to your body, and by stress, you need to understand the physical exercise. This will force the fat burning process, will increase even more the ketones levels, and the insulin will take care of the stored glucose from your blood.

CHAPTER 5: INTERMITTENT FASTING

AND AUTOPHAGY

The concept of intermittent fasting means that you have to fast at regular intervals of the daily routine. Autophagy works tremendously under such circumstances, and with the passage of time, the working length can be achieved mordaciously. However, there are certain techniques that need to be compensated for while you are doing intermittent fasting. They are as follows:

1. THE KETOSIS STATES

It is a state of intermittent fasting in which the body is able to lower down its metabolic rate, and all the saturated fats located in various parts of the body are easily eliminated. You tend to start this while you are at the 12th hour of your body level, and this state forces you to be away from all those bad things that are quite hectic for your body. You become all composed and compassionate in yourself while you are on this diet, and thus, you are all good to come and proceed in the coming.

2. THE RECYCLING OF CELLS

During the second state of the body, the body is able to do the recycling of cells. The cell line is so lenient and efficient in this scenario that you become very effective in this regard. The recycling of cells is an autophagy process and helps to improve the circulation of blood in your holistically. Therefore, the use of autophagy is tremendously very effective for your body to work on, and with this, you are able to make a better transition in your body by all means necessary.

3. THE 54 HOURS SHIFT

By this state, the insulin level has dropped by 54 percent, and you are feeling very relaxed and better in your style. This the hours' shift that helps you to lessen any composed fat on your waistline, and with the passage of time, you are able to be very strong and sustainable in your requirement. Therefore, these three stages are a must to learn states of intermittent fasting, and for anyone who desires to have an autophagy run in it, the 54 hours shift is the best shift for it.

INCORPORATING INTERMITTENT FASTING

In order to incorporate intermittent fasting in you. You have to adopt the following things in yourself.

1. BE PATIENT AND COMPOSED

This means that any diet that has a good number of intakes in it and can deliver a better potential in you with the passage of time, is essential and effective for you. The idea in this scenario is that you have to look for diet and body ideas that can be helpful for you on a coherent level and could engage the best out of you. This might be a little problematic at first, but with the passage of time, you will be able to harness it.

2. ALWAYS LOOK FOR A GREEN DIET

The green diet will help you to pay a better benefit to your body. You will be able to see how the body language is able to incorporate better standings in you, and with the passage of time, you are able to furnish yourself to the next level. Therefore, it is important for you to understand that looking for a green diet for you is the best thing that ever happened to you, and you must incorporate it in the coming time.

INTO YOUR WORKOUT PLAN

The keto diet and the process of autophagy should be incorporated into your workout plan. You must be able to see how the workout is able to make you stand out in front of any issue. You must incorporate physical exercises that could be very effective for your brain and could make you very established in physique as well. Therefore, the incorporation of a workout plan is necessary for you to understand how the body is being moved with possible direction and how autophagy can help to relate in this manner.

CHAPTER 6: PRECAUTIONS TO TAKE REGARDING AUTOPHAGY AND FASTING

Fasting has a lot of advantages. However, fasting is not meant for everyone. To better understand the theory of fasting, let us compare Fasting to a tool (such as an arrow), which can be either used properly or misused. Holding to that, we will use the archery metaphor to explain the effective use and the misuse of fasting/autophagy. A hunter could have different sizes and tips of arrows in his quiver. When he finds an antelope, he will use a sharp wooden arrow, but when he faces a lion or bear, he would go for something stronger: probably an arrow with metallic tips. The point is not to use the wrong method for the right purpose.

WHO SHOULD AVOID FASTING

Pregnant and breastfeeding mothers. Whether you have a child you're breastfeeding or one who is still in your uterus, you need all the calories you can get; both the mother and the infant need to be fed well to stay nourished and healthy.

Underage students and those under the age of 18 should avoid fasting.
Children under the age of 18 are still growing and need all the vital
nutrients and minerals to have healthy growth and development.

Those that are underweight and/or malnourished. If you find it difficult
to tell whether you are malnourished or not, you could ask your
physician or a trusted friend. Those having an eating disorder such as
bulimia are included in this category.

Individuals who have Type-2 Diabetes. Fasting has been used over the
years as a means of reversing the effect of Type-2 diabetes. However,
you still need to consult your physician before beginning a fast.

WHO NEEDS TO BE CAUTIOUS?

Another group of individuals who also need to be cautious is those with
occasional gastroesophageal reflux disease (GERD). Those who fall into
this category need to check with their physician as well if they wish to
fast and must be closely monitored.

There are solid pieces of evidence to prove that GERD could be
aggravated by fasting and the symptoms could become worsened. This
possible worsening is because during fasting, the stomach will be devoid
of food, and there will be nothing which the gastric juice would digest.

Individuals on medications need to be cautious while fasting as the
fasting periods could overlap when such drugs would be taken,
especially those medications that would require you to eat before using
them.

In addition, those on cancer therapy and other medical treatment must
be cautious and should have an in-depth discussion with their physician
before fasting.

CHAPTER 7: INTERMITTENT WATER FASTING

Water is life. No cell in your body can function without it. No living thing on Earth can exist without water's vital essence. Because performance autophagy relates to cell tissue cleansing and renewal, without water, this process would be null and void. The basic human cell is protein, fat, cholesterol, and water. While you begin to increase autophagy through fasting and ketosis, you begin the process of reducing wastes and toxins in the body on a cellular level.

Water will get used to performing all these functions, collecting and disposing of the exhausted materials and compounds. The point of energy is to give life to our experience. The point of water is to give life to that energy. Because water is so significant to the system as a whole, water fasting is a described method of autophagy on account of its ability to enhance autophagic reaction and response.

Timing is everything. Intermittence is a level of time that allows your body to receive ample energy through healthy eating and diet, followed by moments and periods of fasting. This alternating effect brings about effective autophagy, giving space and time to the cells to renew and for the body to gain nutrients; both are necessary for optimal health.

Water fasting is the method by which all food is eliminated slowly over the course of several hours and/or days to allow your body time to gently respond and react to fewer calories. Water is then increased to allow for proper autophagic response and activity. The only thing consumed in water fast is water; however, some vitamins and minerals may be consumed for proper internal balance. Although no calories are ingested, some vitamins and minerals are necessary for the proper function of the cells so that they may do their work during autophagy.

Water is essential; it carries all life and acts as the conduit of all internal functions and performance. Without it, autophagy wouldn't work. Balancing the fast with extra water is key to a healthy autophagic response and brings about greater change, renewal, and deep cellular healing.

CHAPTER 8: COMMON KINDS OF

WATER FASTING

There are many different ways that you can perform a water fast. All these types of fasting will offer you benefits; it's up to you to select one that suits your individual needs, your lifestyle requirements, and your end goal.

1. DRY FASTING

This fast is the most extreme and often called the *Absolute Fast*. The roots of dry fasting are spiritual and consist of foregoing water and food for short periods. We do not necessarily recommend this, as it is really only for very experienced fasters.

2. LIQUID FASTING

This is fasting using only liquids – no food is consumed whatsoever. This can be any liquid or can be more specific as shown by the types of fast that follow.

3. JUICE FASTING

This fast includes some nutritional value just in a pure, or natural, form and is very popular. This is because almost any vegetable, fruit, or juice can be blended with the powerful juicers that are currently on the market.

4. WATER FASTING

This fast may be the oldest of its kind and is thought to provide the greatest physically therapeutic benefit in a shorter period of time because the detoxification process happens quickly. Water fasting is also the easiest type of liquid fasting.

5. MASTER CLEANSE

This is a relatively new method, which is often called the *Lemonade Diet*.

Master Cleanse Recipe

Combine:

- 8 oz purified water

- 2 tbsp lime or lemon juice, fresh squeezed

- 2 tbsp maple syrup, 100% pure

- a dash of cayenne pepper

Recipe yields one 10 oz serving. Drink the mixture anytime through the day, up to 12 glasses daily.

Here are *some tips if you decide that this is the diet for you*:

- If you are prone to hypoglycemia, Master Cleanse is not recommended due to its high sugar levels.

- The night before you plan to start this fast, drink one cup of herbal laxative tea.

- Blend up enough for each day's serving before your first meal, adding the pepper and lemon fresh as you pour each drink, and plan on consuming 6-12 glasses per day.

- Plan on using lemons at room temperature. To best release the juices, roll them, applying firm pressure, back and forth across the countertop right before juicing.

- Don't worry about feeling lightheaded or dizzy. You could be consuming about 650-1300 calories per day from the syrup.

- Drink one cup of herbal laxative tea every evening during your fast.

- After using the Master Cleanse for 10 days, take 3 days for a successful transition back to solid foods. On Day 1, drink several glasses of orange juice throughout the day. On Day 2, eat fresh fruit and drink orange juice and vegetable broth. On Day 3, include fresh vegetables with Day 2's list of food and drinks. Return to a normal diet on the following day.

6. SELECTIVE FASTING

Selective fasting, sometimes known as *partial fasting*, combines liquid fasting with some solid food. It could range from a little bit to a lot based on your needs. You can even choose to combine some of these fasting techniques to fit around you!

CHAPTER 9: WEIGHTLOSS AND WATER FASTING

There have been a number of different kinds of weight loss programs you may have come across in recent times. From choosing weight loss supplements to enrolling for exercise regimes that may seem completely out of place to adapt to a diet that you may believe works well in your favor, weight loss is something you can't get out of your mind when you are overweight. However, when it comes to losing weight, you need to keep in mind that it's not a temporary solution that you should rely on. Relying on these will help you get to the desired weight before you decide to go back to your old habits.

Weight loss is all about changing the way you look at life and incorporating certain techniques that will benefit you in the long run and keep you healthy from within as well. A common misconception with weight is that if you are not overweight, you are healthy. The truth, however, is people who aren't that heavy may also suffer from a number of health conditions because of damaged cells in their body, and this is why you need to consider leading a healthy lifestyle rather than obsessing over weight loss or weight management. Having said that, adapting to autophagy has a number of benefits, and weight loss is definitely one of them. The only difference between the weight loss program that autophagy has to offer versus other weight loss programs is that autophagy benefits you from within.

LOSING WEIGHT FOR THE LOOKS

The most obvious reason somebody wants to lose weight is to look good. When you are a few pounds overweight, your confidence level automatically starts to drop, and a feeling of inferiority starts to seep in. While you should always be confident about the way you look, if you are not happy with your appearance, you should do something to change it.

There are tons of people who start getting depressed because of their weight, mainly because they can't manage to get in shape no matter what they do. The main reason you might not be able to lose weight is because of low metabolism levels. If your metabolism rate is low, no matter how much you diet or starve yourself, you are not going to get in shape. It is important for you to adapt to autophagy so that you start off the process of weight loss and you boost your metabolism rate in order for your body to start burning fat. This is not going to happen overnight, which is why you have to prepare yourself for long-term results. Do not look for shortcuts.

The problem with most weight loss programs today is that they promote weight loss as a trophy for something that you will do for the next thirty days. Simply popping a pill or following a diet plan only for a month to lose weight is the worst thing you can do to yourself. Not only will this affect your body internally, but it will also reflect on your appearance. While some of these weight loss solutions help you to get in shape, they end up giving you horrible skin, tired eyes, and severe hair loss. This is caused because of the lack of nutrients in your system.

If you want to get healthy and you want to do it the right way, you have to give your body time. Autophagy isn't as popular as other quick weight loss solutions because it's not a quick fix. It is a longtime commitment that you have to make, not only so that you look great but also so that you feel amazing from within and you wave goodbye to illnesses.

LOSING WEIGHT TO GET HEALTHY

As mentioned earlier, most weight loss solutions are so that you look great physically, but what you really need is one that makes you healthy from within. One of the most important things you need to understand is that losing weight isn't just about looking great, but also getting healthy at the same time. In order for you to do that, you have to choose something that benefits your body internally as well as externally. The reason autophagy is so great is that it helps with repairing your body from within, and you will also be able to see the results externally.

The main difference between a short-term weight loss program and the autophagy way of life lies in the name itself. A short-term weight loss solution will give you short-term results, and you will eventually end up gaining weight and suffer from a number of health problems. Once you activate autophagy, not only will you start losing weight, but you'll get healthy, and this is essential in order for you to keep illnesses away.

Autophagy helps you to reverse the signs of aging because it repairs the cells in your body, and this keeps a number of age-related diseases away, making it a long-term and effective solution that grows on you. While it's not the easiest weight loss process to get used to, it is something that you will learn to adapt and manage to incorporate for the rest of your life so that you lead a healthy life and focus on being healthy rather than just looking great.

CHAPTER 10: INTERMITTENT FASTING

COULD HELP YOU AGE SLOWLY

One of the biggest benefits of autophagy is seen in the anti-aging effect, which arises when you restrict calorie intake, this makes autophagy possible.

One of the major characteristics of a young organism is a high rate of autophagy. With time, however, autophagy reduces and sets the stage for cell damage. By seeking ways to induce autophagy via fasting, you can slow down aging. We age when there are lots of damaged cells, as well as an inability to recycle old cells.

From the above, it is evident that aging and autophagy seem to be linked. Without enough autophagy in mammals, degeneration of cells follows. This degeneration manifests as aging, which is linked to reduced autophagy. This is why autophagy is an effective tool to mitigate aging.

To understand the relationship between autophagy and aging, a knowledge of how cells replicate is vital. The human body has more than 100 trillion cells (Atkinson, 2018), of which more than 200 billion cells undergo division daily. At times, these cells get sick and worn out, so when they divide, they will produce more sick and weak cells. With time, the higher the number of sick and damaged body cells, the more you age. This is where autophagy comes in, as a means to repair these damaged cells to make them young and healthy again.

We have established autophagy as the internal cellular repair process. In simple terms, autophagy targets old and weak cells and refurbishes them to make them healthy while getting rid of others.

AUTOPHAGY LOWERS RISK OF NEURODEGENERATIVE DISEASE

With time, a man grows; he gets subjected to the disease of the aging brain. However, these ailments might take a while to manifest because of the presence of proteins in the brain cells, protein cells that are not acting right. Autophagy will get rid of this protein, reducing its tendency to accumulate.

For Alzheimer's disease, for instance, autophagy helps get rid of amyloid while it gets rid of α-synuclein in Parkinson's disease. One of the reasons dementia is thought to be related to diabetes is because excessive high blood sugar suppresses autophagy. These make it difficult to cleanse the cells.

AUTOPHAGY IMPROVES SKIN HEALTH

The skin is the largest organ in the body. This makes it susceptible to damage from elements like weather changes, chemicals, light, heat, humidity, and other physical damage. The skin takes a lot from the environment, and it is a miracle that it does not look horrible due to wear and tear. The skin, however, with time, undergoes a lot of damage and toxins, which triggers aging.

Although the body is constantly making new cells, with autophagy you can repair the existing ones, which results in glowing, youthful skin. It is also important to note that skin cells engulf bacteria that are harmful to the body. This explains why it is important to have autophagy as a care mechanism for the skin.

CHAPTER 11: HOW TO FAST

CORRECTLY

Before you think about fasting, you need to know your limits. Fasting isn't something that you just jump headfirst into without any preparation or research. Your experience, health condition, daily nutrition, and the relationship you have with food need to be evaluated before you decide to start fasting.

EXPERIENCE AND DURATION

If you are not experienced at fasting, then I recommend that you don't start with a 21-day water fast on your first attempt. You may also have found some information online that might have painted a rather rosy picture about all the benefits that you can reap by going on an extreme diet like a dry fast.

A juice cleanse is a partial fast, and it gives your body some time to get used to the idea of fasting, so I recommend that you start with a simple form of fasting before you opt for a stringent one. Also, ensure that you are aware of all the possible side effects of a fast before you start one. Start with an easy form of intermittent fasting and make your way up to an alternate day fasting plan.

One of the reasons why you must ease into fasting is to understand the way in which your body responds to fasting. If you know what you can expect, then you are in a better position to deal with issues when they come up. Being prepared for expected challenges makes it easier to fast.

HEALTH

Forget about the saying, "feed a cold, starve a fever." You need to focus on your general health and not just your immediate weight loss goals before you start fasting. If you are fasting as a means to detox your body from a junk food binge, then come up with an alternative or healthy diet plan before fasting.

You must remember that your overall health is more important than anything else that might come your way. If you are on the list of people I mentioned above, then refrain from fasting at all costs. If you don't pay attention to your health, it will land you in a lot of trouble, so please consult your doctor before you start fasting or making any changes to your diet.

NUTRITION AND HYDRATION

Are you wondering what nutrition I am talking about while fasting? You need to understand that your body has a natural inbuilt reserve of certain key nutrients, like fat-soluble vitamins, that help with the regular functioning of the cells when you aren't eating.

You need to ensure that your body has plenty of water-soluble minerals and vitamins while fasting. This means that you need to ensure that your body has sufficient electrolytes within it to function normally. If your body starts running out of these important electrolytes, it will lead to dehydration and will have a negative effect on your body's metabolism.

An essential form of nourishment that your body needs is water. It is not only necessary for transporting nutrients in the body, but it is also important for water removal and the regulation of your body temperature. Water provides a medium within which all other metabolic processes take place, so you need to ensure that your body is thoroughly hydrated at all times.

A lot of fasters tend to experience dehydration because their bodies aren't getting the usual volume of food, and it means that they will need to make up for this deficit. The best way to do this and eliminate any of the negative effects of dehydration is to keep your body thoroughly hydrated.

RELATIONSHIP WITH FOOD

All those who are experiencing any eating disorders or have suffered from any in the past need to avoid fasting until they have overcome those issues. It might seem quite appealing to fast, but it can lead to a relapse of any unhealthy condition.

If you have any history of food abuse or you use food to cope with emotional stress or trauma, then the first thing that you must do is work on developing a healthy relationship with food before you think about fasting. If you don't, then it will only lead to additional stress that is rather unnecessary.

You will learn more about the different tips that you can follow while you are fasting in the coming chapters. Each person has a different response to intermittent fasting. You will never be able to gauge how your body will react to fasting by comparing yourself to the people around you.

You will need to see how your body reacts and make any changes required. What might work for one person might not work for you, and that's perfectly all right. Everyone is different, so the best thing that you can do is to listen to your body. Your body knows what it wants, so learn to listen to it. Also, while you are fasting, you need to take it easy on your exercise regime for a couple of days. Give your body and yourself some time to get used to your new diet.

CHAPTER 12: AUTOPHAGY, KETOSIS, AND FASTING

Autophagy is an important process that restores worn-out cells during starvation and fasting. It is a critical aspect of anti-aging and longevity experienced in caloric restriction. Fasting is one of the most effective methods of increasing autophagy.

Ketosis refers to the metabolic state of high ketone utilization and production. It occurs when your body's glycogen stores are suppressed, and the liver generates ketones that replace glucose. You can experience ketosis during fasting or when under a low carb ketogenic diet.

Ketosis and autophagy support each other even though they are not mutually inclusive. Still, you can be in ketosis without autophagy, and you can experience autophagy without ketosis. It is only that you will see them together because they share similar principles.

DOES AUTOPHAGY NEED KETOSIS?

Here's what controls autophagy and ketosis:

- Autophagy is stimulated under energy deprivation caused by a deficiency of amino acid, fasting, thermoregulation and glucose restriction. In metabolism, you will require little insulin, high AMPK, and low mTOR.

- Ketosis is attained when there is glucose restriction. The main feature that leads to the development of ketone bodies is carbohydrate deficiencies and glycogen depletion. Protein can also lead to carbohydrate synthesis via gluconeogenesis. However, it is secondary and doesn't impact ketosis that much. As a result, you don't need low insulin or low mTOR, although it always happens.

You can experience ketosis while consuming high amounts of mTOR and higher insulin because you consumed something that contains high levels of protein. It will regulate nutritional ketosis and a high level of ketones, but it will inhibit autophagy because of the high nutrient content aspect of mTOR that prevents autophagy.

Autophagy doesn't need ketosis to be stimulated because you can fast for up to 3 days and still not experience ketosis, based on the nature of your keto-adaptation. But remaining in ketosis fulfills most of the prerequisite of autophagy-like low blood glucose, low insulin and lower mTOR. You only need to base it on the period you have been fasting for.

MEASURE KETONES TO DETERMINE AUTOPHAGY

There are no genuine methods to measure autophagy in human beings, but it can be estimated by reviewing the glucose ketone index and the ratio of insulin to glucagon.

Lower insulin to glucagon ratio indicates more ketogenesis, fat oxidation, catabolism, and nutrient deprivation.

A higher ratio of insulin to glucagon indicates more anabolism, increased blood sugar, higher insulin, and nutrient storage.

The glucose ketone index reveals an estimated ratio of insulin-glucagon with a lower score reflecting higher ketosis and more AMPK.

The time it takes before autophagy starts depends on the nutrient status of your body and the availability of specific nutrients, especially glucose and ketones.

If you are not eating a lot of carbs or too much protein daily, then you can expect autophagy to kick in faster than that person who has to burn through those calories first.

AUTOPHAGY ON KETO

Experiencing ketosis while consuming the ketogenic diet can boost the autophagy process and recycle unique proteins via chaperone-mediated autophagy. This can still happen even while eating as long as your carbs and protein remain low.

A ketogenic diet can limit neuronal injury through autophagy and mitochondrial pathways in seizures. It emulates a lot of features of the fasted physiology like mTOR and lowers insulin.

However, the ketogenic diet emulates most of the benefits of fasting and probably helps stimulate autophagy faster than other diets. But for that to succeed, you would require to adhere to the real therapeutic macros of 5% carbs, 70-80% fat, and 15-20% protein. Many people eat a lot of protein and carbs, which is better but it's not going to regulate a constant state of autophagy.

Consuming a low carb ketogenic diet that regulates carbs and doesn't over-do protein is a great basal template for controlling good metabolic health and being ready to get into autophagy faster.

Besides fasting, the therapeutic ketogenic diet that includes some type of intermittent fasting and not more than 2 meals per day is the nearest thing you can get to an autophagy-mimicking diet.

Eating once every day on a keto combined with exercise, consuming autophagic foods, and exposure to other hermetic stressors is one of the most autophagy boosts you can attain while sticking within the 24-hour period. In general, the actual benefits of autophagy start after 24 hours and extend for 3-5 days of fasting.

ARE KETONES THE BEST FUEL FOR BURNING FAT?

If you have ever been to a gas station to pump fuel into your car, you must have seen these three numbers (87-89-93) listed on the pump. But what do they really represent? Maybe someone has ever told you that those numbers represent the rating of something known as octane, which defines the level of compression a fuel can endure before igniting. The higher the octane, the less likely the fuel is to pre-ignite at higher pressures and destroy the engine.

Your body is like a car because it needs fuel to run. Food is your octane, but you can choose the type of fuel to use. You can decide to run on a low octane (sugar) or a high octane (fat). Feeding your body with sugar fuel is likely to cause your body to burst out with fat and be destroyed with chronic disease. On the flip side, fat fuel is highly efficient and will ensure you remain lean.

HOW KETONES ARE GENERATED

Ketones are generated when very little amounts of carbs are consumed, and the body breaks down fats. As a result, it produces fatty acids, which are burned off within the liver through beta-oxidation. Similar to fats, carbs are one of the major food types. But carbs change into sugar when synthesized by the body, which results in obesity and health challenges. Alternatively, the human brain and body prefer ketones as its main energy source because it runs 70 percent more efficiently than sugar.

From an evolutionary perspective, this preference looks sensible. Keeping in mind that carbs were not easily accessible during prehistoric days.

WHY YOU NEED TO MAKE KETONES YOUR MAIN FUEL

The state in which the body processes ketones as its major fuel is known as ketosis. Ketones are produced when the body has an insufficient amount of sugar. When the body is deficient in sugar, you switch to ketosis.

Your body needs the energy to control metabolism. This energy is kept as glycogen or fat. Until your body requires energy, glycogen is stored inside the skeletal muscles and liver. When glycogen is stored in your body, it is changed into sugar when needed. Because it is easier for your body to utilize this energy, you have to use it before it starts to burn fat. In the absence of glycogen, your body will convert stored fat into ketones.

A typical human being has around 600 grams of glycogen inside the body. This is approximately 500 grams in skeletal muscles and 100 grams in the liver.

WHAT FOODS TO EAT TO PRODUCE KETONES

Diet experts have marketed the keto diet because it is effective at burning fat. However, most keto diet resources don't talk about the right foods and nutrients that stimulate cravings. As a result, humans continue to gain weight and grow unhealthy bodies. That is why you need to carefully consider the foods you eat while using ketones to decrease body fat.

It is good to take seafood, pasture-raised eggs, and grass-fed meats because they add protein to your body. Take in carbohydrates from dark green leafy vegetables, and it should make around 5-10% of your diet.

Don't forget to include berries. They are best for low sugar content and high levels of phytonutrients, so you should include blackberries, blueberries, and raspberries. Include a serving of berries daily for its excellent antioxidant protection.

IS IT POSSIBLE TO INDUCE AUTOPHAGY WITHOUT STARVING YOURSELF?

While fasting is the easiest route to turn off nutrient-sensing pathways, but that is not for everyone, as we shall see later. Despite that, most of the physiological responses of a ketogenic diet emulate fasting, and the drop in insulin that happens along with the diet is in part responsible.

If conducted well, the ketogenic diet will trigger the metabolic condition of ketosis where blood ketones have been increased. Beta-hydroxybutyrate, the main ketone body, has been found to activate chaperone-mediated autophagy in vitro. But this was in the context of nutrient deprivation.

CHAPTER 13: HYPERTROPHIC GROWTH

Those that train for strength and sports performance have consistently criticized those who partake in bodybuilding training. Often claiming training for aesthetics is inefficient because optimizing strength, speed, and athleticism should be the primary objective. While there is some truth to this, having more muscle tissue is crucial for many sports and for general health. The key is to train for hypertrophy without sacrificing mobility, speed, body composition, or overall fitness.

Although hypertrophy training is not the most efficient way to build strength, it still offers many benefits to sports performance:

- If two muscles have the same cross-sectional area of muscle fibers, the one with bigger fibers will be stronger.

- Increased GPP (General Physical Preparedness). Hypertrophy training increases work capacity and will allow an athlete to recover faster over time.

- Increased glycogen storage.

- Increased fat oxidation.

- Mass moves Mass. In many sports, having more body weight offers a large benefit, but it is important to make sure this weight is functional muscle instead of body fat.

Studies consistently show that compound barbell exercises are the best when trying to stimulate an anabolic hormone response and increase muscle mass. This is why the primary movements in this program will be the squat, bench, deadlift, and overhead press. There will also be assistance exercises that will all be completed with a barbell as well. The goal with these movements is to focus on moving the maximum load possible while remaining proper technique. On top of building muscle, a byproduct of this program will be an increase in strength. I personally compete in powerlifting and have set personal records coming right out of this program.

I have implemented several key principles to the <u>performance hypertrophy program</u>:

- *Submaximal Loads:* All prescribed training loads in this program will remain under 90% of the 1RM (1 rep max). Many studies show how beneficial the minimum effective dose really is. You can stimulate close to the same effect with a lesser load but also recover much quicker and not inhibit performance on the following training days. Lifting with a maximal load, like in a traditional powerlifting program, does not allow for the amount of training volume this program requires. Also, the risk of injury is greatly decreased when training with weights that are easily lifted.

- *Undulating Periodization:* Undulating periodization adjusts the volume and intensity of each lift within each week. If the program calls for a heavy squat this week, deadlifts will be lighter. This will allow the lifter to lift heavier and recover quicker. Linear periodization, which has been widely used by many for years, is dead. It's outdated and definitely not applicable to high-level athletes.

- *No Weak Links:* The assistance exercises in the program will be variations attacking weaknesses in the athlete's physique. In any athletic scenario, the individual can only perform as well as their weakest link. By attacking these head on, we will correct dysfunction, increase performance, and decrease the risk of injury.

- *Recover, Recover, Recover:* There are only four workout days per week in this program, and that is very important. When focusing on hypertrophy, the recovery periods are more important than lifting. On these recovery days, take the opportunity to focus on mobility and overall health. Lower intensity yoga is highly suggested.

- *Caloric Surplus:* When trying to build muscle, a caloric surplus is essential. A pound of muscle requires an additional 2,500 calories, so make sure to eat enough food. Focus on protein as much as possible.

It must be understood that this program is for intermediate to advanced lifters only. These barbell movements come with a higher risk of injury, so if you are not proficient in these exercises, please seek the help of a fitness professional or look to one of our beginner programs.

CHAPTER 14: LONGEVITY AND AUTOPHAGY

Taking care of your health doesn't have to make you feel like you're doing a chore or restricting yourself. Even if you're not keen on fasting, or if you simply want to opt out of a restrictive diet and eat normally, there are ways to guarantee that you activate autophagy to improve your well-being.

The key is to balance your diet according to your daily needs, and for that, you must choose your foods wisely. In each food category, there are substances that can prevent aging and trigger autophagy. While there aren't specific substances in food that are known to target autophagic regulation, you can fill your plate with a few options that will surely boost the benefits of existing autophagic processes.

Antioxidant-rich foods are an example. Mainly found in vegetables, antioxidants are molecules that function as a defense against free radicals. They can be produced by the body, but diet is a great source and can also stimulate the body to produce a greater amount of these protectors of the body.

It's as simple as following a color code: the more colorful, the more antioxidant-rich foods are. Red-colored foods, such as tomatoes, contain the substance lycopene. It helps to remove a part of the oxygen we breathe called free radicals. They are linked to degenerative processes like cancer and the aging of the body. Fruits still have great antioxidant power, as they protect the body from the harmful action of free radicals. Lycopene has an important anti-aging function in protecting the prostate and cardiovascular system. The substance is always better absorbed by the body along with extra virgin olive oil, which helps in lowering bad cholesterol.

Soy has high levels of isoflavones, vitamins, fibers and minerals, therefore, it has a multitude of benefits: reduces the risk of breast cancer, helps menopausal symptoms and contains effective coadjuvants to prevent prostate cancer and osteoporosis. Yogurt is also another great friend of longevity. It is rich in calcium. The yogurt also has bacteria, the family lactobacillus, which are beneficial to the body, as well as being able to protect the intestinal tract against infections. (*Lv, X., Liu, S. and Hu, Z. 2017*)

Vegetables, broccoli, and cauliflower have nutrients such as the compound sulforaphane, which can destroy carcinogenic substances. Spinach and orange, on the other hand, contain iron and folic acid, which prevents the irritation of blood vessels and consequently heart attacks. It also contains two nutrients that lower your chances of developing blindness. Chestnut and fish, such as salmon and sardines, have omega-3 fat. It lowers the level of bad cholesterol and triglycerides, types of fats that can be produced by the body or ingested through food. Fibers found in cereals, nuts, pumpkin seeds, and sesame seeds also help lower cholesterol. (*Law, B., Chan, W. et al. 2014*)

All these effects are synergistic with autophagy, so it is important to consume a variety of foods rich in antioxidants. Eating a diet rich in antioxidants has been shown to promote health and longevity. In fact, some types of antioxidants have been associated with a 30% reduction in mortality in older adults.

CHAPTER 15: OXIDATIVE STRESS AND

YOUR HORMONES

Aging is a continuous and progressive physiological process, where there's a decline in biological functions, as previously seen. This decline during aging is directly associated with an increased chance of developing neurodegenerative diseases. If you depend on other people to complete simple tasks on a daily basis, for example, you may have a higher risk of developing memory problems or see your cognitive capacities reduced.

There are other psychosocial implications in aging that we are often not aware of and which are determinant in the life of the elderly. A decline in the quantity and quality of social life are inevitable as we age. This factor can exacerbate biological factors that contribute to decline and further aggravate health problems. Thus, we can conclude that aging is a multifactorial process, dependent on genetic factors and individual habits. Habits can increase the susceptibility to develop diseases, and the psychological implications appear as an interdependent factor in aggravating diseases such as neurological pathologies. (*Nixon, R., 2013; Komatsu, M. et al., 2006; Shacka, J., 2008*)

In addition to this gradual loss of the capacity to perform physiological functions and to trigger adaptive responses, there's an increase in functional and structural impairment of different systems, including the central nervous system. One of the hallmarks of aging in the nervous system is the natural formation of senile plaques. These plaques, composed of protein aggregates, were linked to natural cell death and cognitive function deterioration in neuropathologies such as Alzheimer's disease, Parkinson's, amyotrophic lateral sclerosis, among others. Sporadic forms of these diseases make up the majority of observed cases, and their pathological basis is similar. It's still unclear how these factors initiate the neurodegenerative process, as they are heavily interconnected. Studies in molecular biology of aging have identified key cellular changes that can aggravate the existent damage and lead to neuronal death. (*Shacka, J., 2008; Wong, E. and Cuervo, A., 2010; Ghavami, S. et al., 2014*)

Cellular dysfunction due to protein aggregation is related to the damage of the organelles and vesicles traffic in general. Neuronal survival depends on the integrity and functionality of mitochondria. Mitochondria produce energy for the cell and protect the cell from oxidative stress, functioning as a cell quality checkpoint. Cumulative stress as a person ages is involved in early neurodegeneration and undermines this quality control. Thus, the mitochondria become more vulnerable, and the damage caused increases the levels of reactive species, which in turn influence the mitochondria's capacity to produce energy. (*Ghavami, S. et al., 2014; Tsai, S. et al., 2014*)

With aging there is also an increase of ROS related toxicity in the central nervous system, preceding protein aggregation and neuronal loss, as ROS removal mechanisms also suffer damage. We can mention the superoxide dismutase (SOD) and catalase (CAT) systems, which remove superoxide anions and hydrogen peroxide from the cytoplasm. Decreases in metabolic waste removal rates are also linked with an imbalance of neuronal homeostasis.

Changes in protein quality control and apoptotic pathways are also observed. Intracellular degradation processes such as autophagy can be heavily influenced by this gradual change in cellular biodynamics, and vice-versa. Some proteins involved in this pathway play a central role in neurodegeneration. For example, the ULK-1/Beclin-1 complex, involved in the initial phases of autophagocytosis, generate vesicles with a double lipid layer. The equivalent of Beclin-1 in yeast autophagy models is atg6, which participates in yeast's cellular survival mechanisms. A dysfunction in atg6 was proved to induce cancer and neurodegeneration. (*Cai, Y., Arikkath, J., 2016; Ghavami, S. et al., 2014*)

Another important protein in this system is LC3II, which is often used as a marker of autophagy. It was originally identified as a microtubule-associated protein and associates with the autophagosome membrane. LC3I is cytosolic, and LC3II is associated with the autophagic membrane. The detection of LC3I and LC3II is a sensitive marker for distinguishing and studying autophagosomes and is useful for monitoring the state of autophagocytosis since the conversion between LC3I in LC3II correlates with the number of autophagosomes.

As aging progresses, increasing evidence indicates that there is a reduction in the rate of autophagosome formation, maturation, and the fusion of these with the lysosome. Deficiencies in intracellular degradation processes are associated with the formation of protein aggregates characteristic of various neurodegenerative diseases and aging. It has even been shown that cell degradation pathways are impaired in patients suffering from neurodegeneration. More recently, Heng et al. have described the early impairment of the autophagocytic system in Huntington's disease model mice and its possible implication for protein aggregation and cell injury.

Deficiency in autophagy, in particular, is associated with neurodegenerative diseases such as Alzheimer's, Huntington's, Parkinson's, and frontotemporal lobar dementia. The evidence is that the accumulation of autophagosomes in the degenerating brain is associated with the progression of neurological diseases, but the exact relation between the autophagic function of the cell and the appearance of neurodegenerative states still needs to be studied. (*Wong, E. and Cuervo, A., 2010; Komatsu, M., et al. 2006*)

Zheng et al. showed that lysosomal changes appear in the early stages of axonal degeneration, and the maintenance of the function of these organelles could be important in delaying the progression of neurodegenerative diseases. More recently, Ma et al. demonstrated that there is an increase in autophagic activity at the onset of aging in senescence mice. This autophagic activity then decreases with the advancement of age culminating with pathological cellular alterations similar to the characteristics of sporadic Alzheimer's disease.

Disorders in the processes of intracellular degradation may contribute to the deposition of proteins in the brain. In addition, there is evidence that the involvement of the autophagolysosome complex is related to the appearance of Alzheimer's disease characteristics in an experimental model of neurodegeneration. To illustrate the importance of maintaining this system, Cuervo et al. demonstrated that basal suppression of macroautophagy in the brain of mice resulted in protein accumulation and neurodegeneration. In addition, these same authors have demonstrated that α-synuclein can directly damage the lysosomal system.

CHAPTER 16: FINDING THE LONG-TERM AND SHORT-TERM BENEFITS OF AUTOPHAGY

Autophagy helps maintain homeostasis. What is homeostasis? Balanced cellular function in the body is known as homeostasis. Homeostasis, as well as vibrant health, is the result of the p62 protein working its magic during autophagy. As a result of this, all the damaged cells that are accumulated in the body over time are removed, and this creates space for new cells to form. This process does sound good, but how does autophagy benefit you? Here are the benefits of autophagy.

IT CAN BE LIFE-SAVING

It might sound a tad dramatic, but it is quite true. It is scientifically proven. Autophagy's main purpose is life preservation. During times of severe stress like infection or even starvation, this process is kick-started, and it helps optimize the process of repair while reducing damage.

Intermittent fasting activates autophagy and can starve any infectious intruder of glucose. This reduces inflammation so that it is easier for the immune system to take necessary action and help repair the damage that this inflammation and infection has caused. In short, the autophagy mechanism has evolved in such a manner that it helps save energy and repair damage when energy is scarce, but it is also important for the immune system's defense mechanism to fight any illness.

MAY PROMOTE LONGEVITY

Anti-aging benefits certainly sound mythical, almost like a unicorn. Beauty isn't merely skin deep, and it runs deeper. Scientists discovered autophagy during the 50s, and since then there have been several studies that were and are still being conducted to understand the manner in which autophagy improves cellular function and health.

Instead of absorbing any new nutrients, during autophagy, cells tend to replace their damaged parts, get rid of any toxic material within, and start to fix themselves. When the cells in the body begin to repair themselves, they certainly tend to work better, and they act like younger cells.

You might have noticed some people have different biological age and different chronological age. The toxic damage that your body experiences and its ability to repair this situation plays a significant role in these differences.

BETTER METABOLISM

Autophagy is similar to housekeeping service. Not only does it take the trash out, but also it replaces different vital cell parts like the mitochondria. Mitochondria are the powerhouse in a cell that not only burns fat and produces ATP, but is also your body's energy currency. Any buildup of toxins in the mitochondria doesn't just damage cells, and if these cells are destroyed proactively, it helps save future wear and tear of the cells.

Autophagy helps your cells function more effectively and efficiently, and it also helps synthesize new proteins. All this makes your cells quite healthy and this, in turn, improves your metabolism.

REDUCTION OF THE RISK OF NEURODEGENERATIVE DISEASES

Most of the diseases related to the aging of the brain take a long time to develop since the proteins present in and around the brain cells are misfolded, and they don't function like they are supposed to. As mentioned earlier, autophagy helps clean up all these malfunctioning proteins and reduces the accumulation of such proteins.

For instance, in Alzheimer's, autophagy removes amyloid, and in Parkinson's, it removes α-synuclein. There is a reason why it is believed that dementia and diabetes go hand in hand with each other as constantly high levels of blood sugar prevent autophagy from kicking in, and this makes it quite difficult for cells to get rid of the clutter.

REGULATES INFLAMMATION

Do you remember the story of Goldilocks? How she found the perfect bed and the perfect bowl of porridge - that's not too hot or too cold, but just perfect? Likewise, autophagy helps regulate inflammation, and it produces a "Goldilocks" amount of inflammation in the body by either boosting or quelling the response of the immune system according to what your body needs.

Autophagy can increase the presence of inflammation by increasing it when there is an alien body in the body by triggering the defense mechanism of the immune system. Usually, autophagy decreases inflammation from the response of your immune system by getting rid of antigens that trigger it unnecessarily.

HELPS FIGHT INFECTIOUS DISEASES

As I have already mentioned, autophagy helps trigger the immune response as and when necessary. The autophagy mechanism helps get rid of specific microbes that are directly present within the cells like Mycobacterium tuberculosis or viruses like HIV. Autophagy also helps remove the toxins that are produced because of infections, especially any illness that's foodborne.

BETTER MUSCLE PERFORMANCE

Exercise results in slight microtears and slight inflammation of muscles, and this needs to be repaired. The demand for energy increases due to this. The cells in your muscles respond to this by inducing autophagy to reduce the energy that's necessary to use the muscle, eliminate the damaged bits and improve the overall balance of energy to decrease the risk of any future damage.

PREVENTS THE ONSET OF CANCER

Autophagy helps suppress the process that induces cancer like severe inflammation, instability in genomes, and the DNA response to damage. Studies on mice that have been genetically designed to suppress autophagy have shown an increased rate of cancer. As cancer progresses, it might activate autophagy to generate alternate fuel or to even hide from the immune system, but all the research so far has only been on animals and not on human beings.

BETTER DIGESTIVE HEALTH

The cells in the lining of the gastrointestinal tract are at work all the time. A large portion of your feces is cells. When autophagy is activated, your digestive cells have an opportunity to repair, restore, and clear themselves of any junk and reduce or trigger the immune system's reaction as needed.

Any chronic immune response in the gut can not only overwhelm your bowels, but it can also lead to inflammation within, so a chance to rest, repair and clean themselves is important for better digestive health. Autophagy gives your digestive system a much-needed respite from all the work it does.

BETTER SKIN HEALTH

The cells that are exposed in the body are vulnerable to a variety of damage from chemicals, air, light, humidity, pollution, and all forms of physical damage. It's quite a surprise that we don't look worse for wear given all that we expose our skin to. When your skin cells start to accumulate damage and toxins, then they begin to age.

Autophagy helps repair and replace these cells, and it makes your skin look fresh. Skin cells tend to engulf bacteria that can damage the body, so it is quintessential that you support them as they are clearing the clutter.

HEALTHY WEIGHT

Here are a couple of benefits of autophagy that help you maintain a healthy weight.

Short periods of fasting help activate autophagy, burn fat, hold on to muscle mass, and enable you to become lean and fit. It also reduces the chances of unnecessary inflammation that usually leads to weight gain. Autophagy helps reduce the levels of toxins in your body, and when this happens, the cells in your body will not retain a lot of fat.

Autophagy also supports your metabolic efficiency by repairing those parts of the cells that usually create and package proteins and synthesize energy, which is helpful when the cells need to start burning fat to provide energy.

REDUCES APOPTOSIS

Apoptosis is programmed cellular death. When compared to autophagy, apoptosis is quite messy, and it also creates more garbage that needs to be cleaned up. To assist in this cleanup, your body triggers inflammation. The more cells that are repaired, the less effort your body needs to make to clean away old cells and produce new ones.

Renewal of tissues requires less inflammation, so your body starts to use that energy to replace those cells that require constant renewal, like the cells in your digestive system or skin. While some cells need to be renewed regularly, there are some that don't. An increased effort to repair with fewer cleanups is a great combination for your body to function optimally.

CHAPTER 17: BENEFITS OF ONE MEAL A DAY

The popularity of intermittent fasting is increasing every day. One method of IF that is steadily becoming quite popular is the One Meal a Day diet, also known as the OMAD diet. Abstaining from food helps modulate your body's performance, and when you fast for prolonged periods, it has a positive effect on your body and mind.

The OMAD protocol is designed in such a manner that the fasting ratio you need to follow is 23:1. It means that your body will be effectively fasting for 23 hours, and the eating window is restricted to one hour. If you want to burn fat, trigger weight loss, improve your mental clarity, and reduce the time that you spend on food, then eating one meal a day is a brilliant idea.

The OMAD method oscillates between periods of eating and fasting. This method of fasting reduces the eating window more than the other diets. While following this dieting protocol, you need to make sure that you consume your daily calories within one meal and you fast for the rest of the day. OMAD helps you reap all the benefits of intermittent fasting, and it simplifies your schedule as well. The ideal time to break your fast is between 4 and 7 p.m. When you do this, you give your body sufficient time to start digesting the food that you eat before you sleep.

From the perspective of evolution, humans aren't designed to eat three meals per day. As mentioned earlier, our ancestor's bodies were used to functioning optimally even when there was food scarcity. Intermittent fasting protocols like the OMAD tend to kickstart various cell functions in your body that are helpful to improve your overall health. It can be quite intimidating to get started with this method of dieting. There are three simple tips that you can follow to make the transition easier on yourself.

The first thing that you need to do is *slowly cut back on the carbs* that you consume. If you want to optimize the results of this diet and want the least amount of crankiness, then you must limit your carb intake. When you consume a lot of carbs, your body tends to create a stock of glycogen in the body. If there is always some glucose present in your body, then your body will not be able to shift into ketosis. Ketosis is essential to kickstart the process of burning fats. So, if you are trying to start this diet, then it is a good idea to start by slowly cutting back on your carb intake.

You need to *ease your body into getting used to this fasting protocol*. It can be quite difficult to go from eating three meals a day to just one meal a day. You need to ease the transition so that it doesn't feel like you are suffering. A simple way in which you can do this is by slowly getting your body used to the idea of eating fewer meals. So, if you are used to eating three meals per day and tend to snack in between the meals, then the first step is to eliminate all the snacks. Then you can slowly increase the time between the meals and cut down on the number of meals you eat. If you do this, it will be quite easy to follow this diet.

Another simple way in which you can make this diet easier on your body is to consume some caffeine. A morning cup of coffee (devoid of milk and sugar) will make you feel fuller for longer and will keep your hunger pangs at bay.

KEY BENEFITS

WEIGHT LOSS

One of the primary benefits of intermittent fasting is weight loss. Intermittent fasting oscillates between periods of eating and fasting.

While fasting, your calorie intake reduces naturally, and it helps you lose weight and maintain it as well. Apart from that, it also stops you from indulging in any form of mindless eating. Whenever you consume food, your body converts the food into glucose. The glucose that it needs immediately is converted into energy, and the rest is stored within the body in the form of fat cells. Not all the food you consume is converted into energy. So, all the unused energy is stored as fat within your cells. When you start to skip meals, your body will reach into its internal stores of energy. Once your body starts to burn fats to provide energy, it automatically starts the process of weight loss. Also, most of the fat is usually stored in the abdominal region. If you want to lose fat from your abdominal region, then this is the best diet for you.

SLEEP

Obesity is rampant these days. In fact, it is a major health problem that humanity is suffering from. The primary cause of obesity apart from terrible lifestyle and food choices is the lack of sleep. Intermittent fasting regulates your circadian rhythm and encourages a better sleep cycle. When your body is sufficiently rested, it is capable of burning fats effectively. A good sleep cycle has several physiological benefits, like an increase in your energy levels and an overall improvement in your mood.

RESISTANCE TO ILLNESSES

Intermittent fasting assists in the growth as well as the regeneration of cells. Did you know that the human body has an internal mechanism for repairing all the damaged cells? Well, think of it as internal housekeeping that ensures that all the cells in your body are performing optimally. When you follow the protocols of intermittent fasting, it improves the overall functioning of your cells. So, it directly helps improve the natural defense mechanism in your body and increases the resistance to diseases as well as illnesses.

A HEALTHY HEART

Burning up all the stored unnecessary fats in the body helps improve your cardiovascular health. The buildup of plaque in the blood vessels is referred to as atherosclerosis. Atherosclerosis occurs when fat deposits start building up in the blood vessels, and it is the primary cause of different cardiovascular diseases. The endothelium is a thin lining present in the blood vessels, and a dysfunction of this lining causes atherosclerosis. Obesity is one of the main reasons for the build-up of plaque in blood vessels. Stress, as well as inflammation, worsens this problem. Intermittent fasting helps reduce and remove plaque deposits and helps tackle obesity. So, if you want to improve the health of your heart, then this is the best diet for you.

A HEALTHY GUT

Did you know that your gut is the home for several millions of microorganisms? These microorganisms are helpful and are essential for the optimal functioning of the digestive system. These microorganisms are known as microbiome. The gut microbiome is necessary for a healthy gut. A healthy digestive system helps with better absorption of food and improves the functioning of your stomach. So, a simple diet change can help you improve your gut's health.

TACKLES DIABETES

Diabetes is a terrible problem. In fact, it is right alongside obesity as one of the leading health concerns these days. Diabetes is also a primary indicator for the risk of the increase of different cardiovascular diseases, like heart attacks and strokes. When the level of glucose is alarmingly high in the bloodstream, and there isn't sufficient insulin to process the glucose, it causes diabetes. When the body starts developing a resistance to insulin, it is quite difficult to regulate the sugar levels in the body. Intermittent fasting reduces the problem of insulin sensitivity and effectively helps tackle and manage diabetes.

REDUCES INFLAMMATION

Whenever your body notices an internal problem, it powers up its natural defense mechanism - inflammation. Inflammation in moderate amounts is desirable and helpful. However, it doesn't mean that all forms of inflammation are good. Excess inflammation causes various health problems like arthritis, atherosclerosis and neurodegenerative disorders. Any inflammation of this form is known as chronic inflammation. Chronic inflammation is quite painful, and it can restrict your body's movements.

PROMOTES CELL REPAIR

When you start fasting, the cells in your body engage themselves in the process of waste removal. Waste removal refers to the process of breaking down dysfunctional cells and proteins. This process is known as autophagy and is quintessential for the upkeep of your body. Do you like accumulating waste in your home? Similarly, it is important to ensure that your body doesn't start collecting any toxic wastes. Autophagy is the natural way of getting rid of all unnecessary things from your body. Autophagy protects the neurons in your brain from any cell degeneration. It not only protects the neurons but also prevents them from excitotoxic stress. All this helps the brain replace the damaged cells and replace them with healthy new cells. When your body does this naturally, it improves the health of your brain. Autophagy also increases the lifespan of cells and promotes longevity.

IMPROVES MEMORY

Intermittent fasting also helps improve your ability to learn and retain things. Improving your memory is one of the best protective measures against neurodegenerative diseases. A diet that restricts the intake of calories helps improve your memory.

REDUCES DEPRESSION

Dealing with any mood disorder can be quite tricky. Medication isn't the only means to deal with such disorders. A healthy diet that doesn't fill your body with unnecessary calories leads to an overall improvement in mood. Not just mood, but it also improves your mental clarity and promotes alertness.

CHAPTER 18: FOODS THAT BOOST AUTOPHAGY

Following are some of the foods that stimulate autophagy:

GINGER

Ginger is a food that stimulates autophagy ghastly and makes things come close in an effective manner.

GREEN TEA

Green tea is the best drinking lot that can help you to be lean and adopt autophagy in you. It has some herbs and essential ingredients that are designed to give better illustrations to the people. The green tea is easy to mix and can be capitalized easily in the coming time. The green tea requires no such working in the products and can be available in every possible direction

REISHI MUSHROOMS

Reishi mushrooms can be easily accepted in the world timings, and these mushrooms could be made out of nowhere. The mushrooms make the body language more lenient in its desire, and with the passage of time, the people are able to learn a lot from its core and construct. The constructs of the mushrooms need to be identified with the passage of time, and they are best to carry out an autophagy product.

TURMERIC/CURCUMIN

Turmeric is a regimental disease that could be very healthy and compatible with autophagy. It does not require a lot of work for its process, and it could easily bring the concept of better regulations in the time. Therefore, turmeric and curcumin are the best details looking forward to the people in the society.

Our bodies can detox themselves through natural processes in the livers, kidneys, skin, and bowels and through autophagy. However, we can also take special steps to detox ourselves through our diets and other lifestyle changes. This chapter is dedicated to the reasons why you might want to consider taking further steps to detox yourself.

Detox diets have earned a reputation of being based upon frivolous pseudoscience, but detoxing is an incredibly important process in our body. Our health is assaulted from all angles by toxins and pollutants, everything from caffeine and alcohol to air pollutants from industrial waste, car exhaust, and cigarette smoke. Most of the things we eat, even foods we consider healthy, have small amounts of toxic substances within them. Yet, we can also allow toxins to enter our bloodstream through the skin and through the air that enters our lungs. Regardless of their source, our body regularly needs to deal with all the nasty compounds and chemicals that end up in the body, otherwise, we can face corresponding nasty health consequences.

In the body, the liver and the kidneys are the organs responsible for dealing with toxins in the body. The kidneys filter toxins from the blood, whilst the liver breaks down toxins into substances that can be used by the body or passed without trouble. If the kidneys and liver are burdened with too many toxins or if they are not kept in good shape through a healthy lifestyle, they can be unable to deal with all the toxins in the body. This can cause a huge array of problems, anything from fatigue and general feelings of being unwell to bloating and digestive problems and even liver disease.

Most detox diets are aimed at eating lots of foods that help keep the liver and kidney in tip-top shape, but there are also many other methods to keep these crucial organs healthy. Drinking lots of water – at least 6 to 8 glasses per day – allows any waste products of the liver and kidneys to easily pass through the body. Likewise, you should avoid smoking and second-hand cigarette smoke, which contains over 4,000 different chemicals, including 43 cancer-causing carcinogens.

Eating too much sugar also makes your liver unhappy. By now everyone knows how consuming too much sugar can contribute to diabetes and the various health issues associated with weight gain, but the effects of sugar on the liver remain an enigma to most. The liver has a very limited ability to metabolize sugar, with some dieticians suggesting that anything more than 6 teaspoons of added sugar is excessive. Any sugar that the liver cannot break down is stored as fat, and a build-up of fat in the liver can lead to a condition called fatty liver disease.

Fatty liver disease, in turn, can lead to more serious conditions as bodily pain, fatigue, weakness, and cirrhosis of the liver. Most people who are overweight or obese are at increased risk of fatty liver disease, and they may be suffering from the condition in its early stages when there are few explicit symptoms.

Caffeine is another common toxin that the body has to deal with regularly. Caffeine is commonly associated with coffee, but it is also present in most fizzy drinks, chocolate, and energy drinks. The liver interprets caffeine as a foreign chemical, and it is broken down through a special pathway in the liver that deals with manmade and unfamiliar substances, which includes most medication. For this reason, heavy caffeine consumption should especially be avoided when also taking certain drugs, especially pain relief chemicals such as acetaminophen.

Moderate caffeine consumption isn't dangerous or even unhealthy, with some studies suggesting it has numerous benefits on the body. Nonetheless, for the purposes of cleansing the body of toxins and giving the liver a period of relief, it's best to avoid this energy-booster or at least cut down on your silent addiction.

Good liver health can also be maintained by eating a diet rich in antioxidants, which aid in processing the waste products of toxins. Common antioxidants include vitamin C, vitamin E, beta-carotene, and zinc. Foods which are rich in antioxidants include dark chocolate, legumes, blueberries, red grapes, nuts, dark green veg, orange vegetable, and green tea.

You can also help detox by eating organic food whenever possible. Non-organic foods are free from pesticide residue that may be left on non-organic foods. Many pesticides can build up in the human body and may be dangerous in noticeable concentrations. Eating organic, however, isn't always possible, practical, or affordable, so sometimes it may be necessary to compromise. In general, if you eat the outer surface of grown food, it's more important that it is organic. Fruit such as strawberries, apples, grapes, cherries, and leafy greens should preferably be organic, whereas with fruit or veg with peel it is less important (such as bananas and onions). The easiest way to detox your body is always to avoid toxins in the first place!

There is also a detox method you might not expect; getting more sleep. The western world has an embarrassing relationship with sleep. Sleep is vital for our well-being in dozens of different ways – it's where we rest our minds and rejuvenate our bodies. Yet all too many people resent their need to sleep and try to cheat themselves out of an hour or two every night. This can take a serious toll on well-being.

In terms of detoxing and cleansing the body, most of the detox process occurs during sleep. In the resting state of sleep, your body is free to use resources and act in ways it simply can't when you are awake. For example, one of the main purposes of sleep is to filter toxins out of the brain, toxins which naturally as a side effect of being awake. The filtering system is called the lymphatic system, and it is thought to be 10 times more active during sleep than during wakefulness. During sleep, numerous other metabolic processes take part, such as those which occur in the liver and are inhibited whilst active.

Whilst it might be rather obvious, it is also worth mentioning that you can prevent toxins from getting into your system by avoiding places and environments where there are toxins present. Exhaust fumes, second-hand smoke, and low air quality from industrial pollution are the main culprits, but depending on your location and career you may come into contact with many other types of toxins such as chemical residue from working in a factory, for example.

You can also aid the detox process by taking certain supplements, most notably milk thistle. Milk thistle is a small plant that grows in Mediterranean regions. It can be used as an herb, and it also goes by the names Mary Thistle or Holy Thistle. Milk thistle is a popular natural choice for helping treat liver conditions such as cirrhosis or jaundice, and it is also a staple of the detox community.

The active ingredient in milk thistle is called silymarin, and it has powerful anti-inflammatory properties as well as being an anti-oxidant. Research on silymarin is still progressing, and it's not entirely clear how it affects the body. Some studies have suggested that silymarin can aid liver function in individuals who have been exposed to industrial toxins, such as xylene, and there is evidence to help it also improves type 2 diabetes and lowers cholesterol.

Finally, you can also try a temporary cleansing diet. Ultimately, our body needs the right materials to detox, and as you might now understand, our regular diets don't give us enough resources to work with. You can rectify this by trying a cleansing diet intended to give your body a huge boost of all the vitamins, minerals, and good stuff it needs to cleanse itself.

Of course, ideally, a healthy, balanced diet will help the body cleanse itself over time and be exposed to fewer toxins. However, whether it's due to personal fault or factors beyond our control, we can't always consume a perfectly healthy diet. It might just be too pricey, we might not have the time, or we might constantly be around other people who influence or control our eating habits.

Therefore, as a temporary solution or as a compromise, you can periodically embrace a cleansing detox diet. These types of diets aren't intended to be a permanent change to your eating patterns, and you shouldn't follow them for any period longer than 1-week. However, with that being said, they can give your body a reprieve to repair and rejuvenate itself, a benefit that can last for a few weeks or months before being required once more.

There are many different types of cleansing and detox diets, most of which involve consuming a large amount of fruit, vegetables, and calorie-free drinks. Try one out for a week and see how you feel afterward!

EAT PROBIOTICS!

If you decide to detox, it might seem like the list of prohibited foods is huge. However, there are still many great choices for a detox diet, and you should still find that you can eat a diverse and tasty diet during your detox and body cleanse.

In particular, *probiotics* are a good choice. Probiotics are a group of foods that contain 'good' bacteria that promote a healthy gastrointestinal ecosystem. As you may know, your gut contains tens of thousands of different bacteria, some of which can benefit your health, some which cause harm, and some which have little impact. The health of the bowels is increasingly understood to be crucial to human health, with some studies suggesting that the flora of the gut influencing how many nutrients and calories you absorb from your food and even contributing to mood swings and depressions. In fact, probiotics have also been argued to help prevent diarrhea, gut disease and improve eczema, although the support for these claims is controversial.

There are many different probiotic foods, including yogurt, sauerkraut, miso soup, kefir, sourdough bread, and tempeh, all of which are considered healthy detox-friendly foods, at least when eaten in moderation. Probiotics can also be found as a supplement, although if you decide to take a specific probiotic supplement it's worth further researching what the proposed benefits are – there are many different types of probiotic supplement with all of the different supposed effects.

CHANGING YOUR EATING HABITS

Whether you are attempting a detox diet or trying to fast, you are not only working against your natural instinct to eat but any habits and emotions that revolve around food. You might eat when you are tired to give you a boost in energy, binge to perk up your mood or make poor choices just out of routine or mindlessness. Regardless of your reasons for a detox diet or a fast to work, you need to control how you interact with food.

Start by thinking about your current habits. Are you an emotional eater? Do you like to reward yourself with food? The first stage to overcoming these habits is simply recognizing them and being honest with yourself. It's better to admit your faults rather than to pretend that they don't exist; they'll be there regardless.

By acknowledging how you interact with food you can anticipate and prepare for any temptations that occur during your fast or detox. By depriving yourself of food or by forcing yourself to eat a cleansing diet, you will encounter these feelings, and they will probably be stronger than they usually are.

Learn to challenge your feelings and your thoughts. Are you really hungry? Do you really need to give up on your fast? Isn't there an alternate more productive way to deal with your emotions? Try meditating or doing some activity, such as walking your dog or tackling a task you've been putting off. By engaging with an activity you consider positive you'll feel much better afterward, and the emotions that were bothering you will dissipate.

Also, learn to just sit and be comfortable with your feelings. Instead of shying away from the emotional pain that might be driving you to binge eat, or simply the lack of motivation to continue, take a moment to pause in your day and explore these feelings. Are they strong or weak? How do they affect your thought patterns? How are these feelings affecting your body – can you explore where these feelings are actually occurring? The more you learn to delve into these feelings instead of running away, the more mundane they will become and the less influence they will have over you.

You should also make an effort to be mindful of your eating patterns, in both a detox diet and an eating pattern that involves fasting. You might find that you gorge on your food without truly considering or tasting it, or when you come home from work you automatically start browsing around in the fridge for something to snack on. By trying to be more aware of your interactions with food, you can help manage temptations and habits that urge you to eat.

Finally, try to think positively about your detox diet or fast. Studies have shown that it's easier to change your habits by developing positive habits rather than breaking negative habits. Or in other words, instead of thinking 'I want to stop feeling so lethargic and bloating, it's better to think 'I want to be successful in my detox diet.' These two thoughts might relate to the same goal, but the latter has a much more positive vibe to it, which also makes it easier to strive towards.

DEALING WITH OTHER PEOPLE

Many people won't appreciate the benefits of fasting or a detox diet. You can cite a hundred different studies or try to explain your motivations as logically and clearly as possible, but people might still sneer or disregard what you are doing.

As a result, it's best to consider carefully who you talk about your diet. Do they need to know? Does it bother you if you don't have their approval? It might not be a big deal if someone doesn't accept your diet, but it can still make your life easier if you are not listening to snide comments or objections every time you are around them.

You can always find support online or a detox and fasting community nearby to talk to. These people will understand you and be more welcoming. Of course, you may be fortunate to be surrounded by friends and family who are considerate, or at the very least, appreciate what you are doing is important to you.

If you have to tell people, just try and be as clear and reasonable about the discussion as possible. Laying a strong foundation for why you are doing a fast or detox diet will help people accept it; if your first explanation is watertight, people will find it hard to object, yet if you explain yourself poorly, you'll be dogged by criticism throughout.

CHAPTER 19: CIRCADIAN RHYTHMS AND AUTOPHAGY

Whether you're a night owl or an early bird, getting a good night of sleep goes beyond just improving your mood. Sleep has implications in nearly every system in the body: it boosts cardiovascular health, helps to lose weight, improves your memory, lower stress levels, and is crucial to help the immune system battle infections. During the night, the body goes into "repair mode" and starts cleaning the damage done to the cells during the day, especially in the nervous system. (*Altun, A. and Ugur-Altun, B. 2007; Xie, L. et al. 2013*)

Neurons in the brain oversee all functions in the body, firing electrical impulses, ordering hormone release to regulate your metabolism, and processing external stimuli. This extreme cellular activity causes metabolites and toxins to accumulate inside neurons, namely adenosine, a molecular byproduct of ATP degradation. When adenosine levels rise in the brain, the neuronal function can be impaired. In fact, many neurodegenerative diseases - like Alzheimer's and Lewy body dementia – as well as psychiatric and mood disorders can be linked with poor sleep. (*He, Y. et al. 2016; Ma, D. et al. 2012*)

Sounds familiar? A decrease in autophagy levels is also associated with neuropathies, where astrocytes are unable to remove and degrade accumulated proteins in their lysosomes and avoid neuron destruction, and there are reports that link sleep and autophagy as essential processes for tissue housekeeping and metabolic regulation. In 1970, a series of microscopy studies pointed out that the number of autophagosomes in mice cardiomyocytes, hepatocytes, pancreatic and renal cells varied throughout the day, in a similar fashion to the circadian rhythm. (*Ma, D. et al. 2012*)

In mammals, sleep and metabolism are regulated by the suprachiasmatic nucleus (SNC), which is responsible for establishing the circadian rhythm, a 24-hour cycle in which many biological parameters – from blood sugar levels, hormonal concentrations, to feeding signals – vary in distinct diurnal patterns and are prevalent in tissues with high metabolic activity.

At the same time, gene expression in the liver, SCN, and other tissues involved in metabolism also vary, especially for genes that participate in glucose and lipid metabolism. Bmal1 and Rev-erbα expression, in particular, was significantly increased and was later found that it happens along with a peak in autophagic flux. Bmal1 knock-out mice were diagnosed with an impairment in gluconeogenesis and hypoglycemia that increased at night, resulting from an impairment in autophagy.

Cyclic activation of autophagy and its respective regulation genes is therefore considered to be a cellular response to changes in metabolic gears, and if it stops functioning correctly, it can increase the risk of many diseases that were already described. For example, mice that were engineered to express symptoms of Alzheimer's disease showed a cyclic pattern of beta-amyloid protein aggregation, based on how fragmented their sleep cycle was. Autophagy cycles were particularly altered in the hippocampus, the first structure to be affected by a lack of sleep – often leading to memory loss. (*Maiese, K., 2017; Hastings, M. and Goedert, M. 2013*)

Additionally, melatonin levels were altered in mice with sleep deficits, affecting how mTOR regulation of aging and neurodegeneration occurred. Melatonin is the main hormone to regulate sleep cycles and can be severely repressed if we don't keep a regular sleep schedule. (*Merenlender-Wagner, A. et al. 2013*)

CHAPTER 20: SLEEP OPTIMIZATION

Modern society promotes a lifestyle that does not allow for normal circadian rhythms. The use of alarms to wake us up before a shift, artificial lights at our homes that prolong the daylight period in circadian cycles, and using electronic devices before going to sleep are factors that greatly influence our sleep cycles. Endogenously, our melatonin levels are regulated by light/darkness levels, and exposure to longer cycles contributes to a dramatic shift in its production.

Observational studies with populations of the Amazon jungle have confirmed these suspicions. These populations had no access to electric light, and their sleep cycles were longer by 30 minutes than occidental populations. This phenomenon is becoming even more common in an increasingly technological, nocturnal, and competitive world, a byproduct of our working schedules.

This hypothesis takes particular relevance in countries that have flourished technologically in the post-war, as in the case of South Korea and Japan. South Korea is highly competitive in academic and work terms, where sleep time is shortened when economic circumstances so dictate, being inversely correlated with time spent at work and salary.

However, these trends have mixed standards in many countries, with varying literature within the same country. These contradictory data do not, in any way, refuse the idea that chronic sleep deprivation has a high prevalence in adults. Any adult aged 25 to 64 years old requires on average 7 to 9 hours of sleep per day, but, according to the CDC, about 34.8% of American adults sleep less than 7 hours a day and have a clearly deficient sleep time with cumulative negative effects. In addition to this, there has been a decline in the sleep hours that children and adolescents get in the past decades. Dollman et al. verified a decrease of about 30 minutes in their daily sleep schedules between 1985 and 2004 in Australian children aged 10 to 15 years. This pattern has been identified in other nations such as Japan, Switzerland, and Iceland. These findings may have some clinical relevance in the appearance of certain pathologies such as hyperactivity disorder with deficit attention, as some differences were observed across studies with children living with this pathology – mainly a shorter sleep duration, increased latency period, patterns of movement during sleep - relative to healthy children.

It is known that most of these changes affect people at an endocrinological level, especially when they only a few hours of sleep per day. Serum levels of cortisol and ghrelin rise and make a considerable increase in appetite and the risk for diabetes or obesity, cardiovascular diseases. There are also consequences for the immune system, where people that sleep less than 6 hours a day can have a decrease or increase in immunological activity, meaning that they are more sensitive to infectious diseases.

Problems related to sleep are also an additional risk factor for accidents at work and for road accidents. To this end, in attention, concentration, increased reaction time, distraction, stress, and irritability. In 2003, a study involving more than 7000 workers from several Dutch industries showed that workers with high rates of fatigue were 70% more likely to be involved in work-related accidents, compared with workers reporting low levels of fatigue, with many of these accidents resulting in fatalities.

If we dive deeper into this knowledge, we can see that biological rhythms exist in all living organisms and regulate many functions, from physiological and mental processes. The grouping of these patterns make up our chronotype, or our individual preference to rest during the day. The disruption of these rhythms is one of the aspects present in depressive syndromes, with many documented setbacks in patients with major depressive disorders, bipolar disorders, and seasonal affective disorders.

In recent decades, a new line of thinking linked the appearance of these disorders with deregulation in autophagy, and that just like we're used to taking the trash out late at night, cells initiate their clean-up process at specific times of the day. For example, researchers have found that mice expressing Alzheimer's disease and that were sleep-deprived for a few days showed higher levels of beta-amyloid, a protein that accumulates in the brain of patients diagnosed with this disease. One of the structures that were more affected by a change in sleep cycles was the hippocampus, which is a tiny bean on our brain that helps us remember facts and things that happen to us during the day. Neurons inside the hippocampus had difficulties starting autophagy, and this sudden block made them less capable to fight back the formation of beta-amyloid.

In any cell, autophagy happens like a dance, in a rhythmic manner, and this dance is choreographed not only by sleep cycles. Metabolism and sleep go hand in hand when it comes to regulating our biological clock. Some metabolic syndromes are caused by terrible sleeping habits, leading to weight gain, hormonal diseases, and cardiovascular diseases. This happens because there are genes that are extremely sensitive to these changes, and they happen to be associated with metabolic processes. Screening of liver, neuronal, and muscular tissues showed that their genetic expression varies according to the time of day and sugar levels, with bmal1 and Rev-erbα being the most altered in their expression. Surprisingly, so did autophagy levels.

As researchers dived further into this rabbit hole, they found that mice with low Bmal-1 levels had more chances of becoming hypoglycemic during the day, and why? Because they couldn't activate autophagy. It was a breakthrough when they found that there was a cycle behind this process and that autophagy was present in higher levels after the mice were fed and lowered at night before they went to rest. The same happens to us. Ever wondered why you feel extremely tired at night? That's your circadian clock working and signaling your body to rest and digest: you are fed, and you are ready to start repairing your body with a good night's sleep. Autophagy is shut down at this time as stress levels go down.

But wait, isn't autophagy supposed to help us repair our bodies? Of course, but autophagy is not a major regeneration mechanism when we sleep. Autophagy is like insurance we have on our cells during the day, which helps them fight back all the damage and stress they take. Nevertheless, it is important to have a good night's sleep, as not to disrupt your autophagic cycles. If you are having trouble keeping your eyes shut at night, don't lose sleep over it, and check out the tips below to have a healthy sleep cycle.

CONCLUSION

To conclude the book, you have to be very careful about the diet intakes that you do throughout your routine. You need to be curious about every calorie that goes into you. You have been provided with all the reasons in this book about the process of autophagy. Autophagy can give you a healthy pH. and can avert any harmful stroke of acidity in the body. Acidity can be dangerous in profuse accumulation of fats, rise to inflammatory disease, the rupture in many digestion organs, and having a rusted metabolism that does not work in the flow. On the contrary, autophagy can give you a fresh intake of all healthy diets that can be very healthy and caring for you. These diets are present in all formats.

They are in breakfast recipes, the dinner recipes, the lunch recipes, the smoothies, and the sweat desserts that can up-satisfaction in your mouth. You do not have to be an expert in medicine to know which diet to follow when. You just have to know the diet intake of your own body and see how you are able to cater to the plight of diseases. You must not be able to compound yourself with the attack of acidity but must have the courage to use these diets and recover at the earliest.

These diets have everything in their DNA. They have the minerals, the enzymes, the protein, the amino acids, and whatnot. Green refluxes along with curing liquids are present in these diets, and they come in all whims and fancies of the diet expression. There is no rocket science behind their creation, and one has to be very intelligent while creating them. You can also follow this book and will get a splendid amount of results in no time. It is available at an affordable price.

Try your best to avoid any acidic diet at all costs, even if it gives you a great amount of relish. The idea is fats and minerals are very delicious, but they come with devious outcomes of fat accumulation and strengths. You need to understand that long aging is only possible if you have a balanced diet intake, and this diet can be only an alkaline one.

To make conclusive remarks of the book about the benefits of an alkaline diet first and foremost is the sheer activeness that a person tends to achieve while he is eating an alkaline diet. He feels healthy and looks healthy and wants to be doing a lot of things while he has an alkaline diet. He can think properly and can get rid of inflammatory diseases that can cause him suffering. He has a strong discipline that can be navigated in any way possible, and thus, he is the next big thing for his users. Also, the longevity of life in this scenario and truly, autophagy can do a lot of wonders for the individual. Therefore, autophagy has a lot to do with the fitness and active-ness in the human body.

Furthermore, if you want to look green and fresh on your face, then autophagy can be very helpful in this regard. Studies show that autophagy is very popular in making a healthy face for you. The number of herbs and breakfast recipes you have for yourself up-bring a good amount of freshness on your face as well on your skin. Thus, autophagy is very crucial for having great skin and face.

You are able to get a lot of chronic pains in your body due to many reasons. You get to the bottom of any problem; you solve it and end up having chronic pain in your body. Chronic pain refers to any tertiary amount of pain in your body, and you are able to get to the harmfulness of it in no time. Therefore, chronic pain is the most devastating headache that you can get, and the only effective cure for it is the alkaline diet. Yes, autophagy is very important for you to maintain as the blood level minimizes when lemon or other alkaline water is induced in the body. So, this is another benefit of autophagy, and it does not matter if you are a walker, a boxer, or even a corporate worker, you must have autophagy in you if you wish to give all that you crave.

In the end, we will only assure you good health and being a beginner, you must waste any further time and order this book in a jiffy. Because health is wealth, nobody became rich while being lazy and stubborn. This book is all that you need, and you must get it at all costs.